M000095700

## Jean Antonello, RN, BSN

Author of the INTERNATIONAL BESTSELLER
*How to Become Naturally Thin by Eating More*
and Creator of the Naturally Thin® Program

# NATURALLY THIN

## *LASTING WEIGHT LOSS WITHOUT DIETING*

Includes the 31-Day Quick Start Plan

Book Cover Design Art Director: Joan Holman

Visit the Naturally Thin website at www.naturally-thin.com

Library of Congress Control Number: 2017909908

ISBN: 978-0-9989477-0-9 (paperback)
ISBN: 978-0-9989477-1-6 (ebook)


Published by Heartland Book Company
3013-13th Terrace NW
St. Paul, Minnesota 55112
612-325-1860

# ACKNOWLEDGMENTS

I especially thank the determined individuals who have applied the principles in this book and have shared their stories of recovery. Their experiences have inspired and encouraged me to continue to teach and write on this subject. Their recoveries have also been a source of hope for the myriads of people still searching for a way out of dieting and disturbed eating patterns—hope for a normal relationship with food, enjoyable, sustainable exercise, Lani Muelrath, Kim Taylor, and Noel Minneci.

I also thank the many crusaders in the field of diet and nutrition, including researchers, physicians, nurses, dietitians, trainers and filmmakers, whose dedication to improving how we eat and think about our diets is clarifying this complicated issue in our country and around the world. I am also indebted to the individuals I have met who personally strive to improve their diets as we learn more about food from new research. Their input has been uniquely helpful. There is a movement in our country, and it is growing to be sure.

Dedicated to Skip Billey

friend
counselor
believer

John 6: 28-29

# TABLE OF CONTENTS

# PREFACE

Readers familiar with my previous books, *How to Become Naturally Thin by Eating More, Breaking Out of Food Jail,* and *Naturally Thin Kids,* are aware of the basic concepts here. *Naturally Thin: Lasting Weight Loss without Dieting* reflects the **Naturally Thin® Program** described in my other books. My purpose in writing a current edition, including the overlap of information, is to educate ever more people who are still confused by the flawed promise of traditional dieting, and there are millions. As time goes on, I hear from more and more ex-dieters and former victims of eating disorders who have found lasting deliverance from food, weight, and eating obsessions because of the principles described in this book. As increasing numbers recover and share how their lives have been transformed by this information, I have hope that, through this book, many others like them will find freedom too.

Losing weight—
Oh rapture gained!
A smaller size,
The thrill it brings—
The vow and how
To go about
Are clear as day

But then the plan
It comes undone.
I lose the loss
That I had won.
So once again
I'm losing weight
Oh rapture gained!

Jean Antonello, 2015

There is a principle which is a bar against all information, which is proof against all arguments, and which cannot fail to keep a man in everlasting ignorance—that principle is contempt prior to investigation.

Source unknown

It ain't what you don't know that gets you into trouble. It's what you know for sure that just ain't so.

–Mark Twain

# Introduction

Virtually every dieter who starts yet another diet is convinced that "this diet" is different. "This diet" includes a weight-training program and aerobics. This diet involves psychological counseling to help you understand the reasons behind your overeating. This diet eliminates food groups that are the culprits in weight gain. This diet promises to magically curb your appetite and cravings so you can stay with small portions. This diet allows you to eat sweets and all your favorite foods so why would you ever want to go off this diet? This diet makes you lose weight so fast that you'll be inspired to stay with it forever. This diet is nationally televised with a full time built in trainer, nutritionist, and cameras all over your house to catch you cheating. This diet is scientifically formulated by doctors and researchers who know what overweight people need to do because they've proved it in laboratory rabbits. This diet is based on decorating schemes, genetics, blood type, body type, eye color, glove size, movie preference, head circumference, and kindergarten art.

Yet, in spite of all these claims and the faith they inspire, diets do fail, most of the time. Statistically, all diets, of every ilk, fail 95 percent of the time. So why do people keep dieting? And why do medical professionals continue to recommend that their patients keep dieting? They do this because there is a logic behind diets that they can't shake, and they don't know what else to do.

All traditional diets have one important thing in common—a prescription for the intake of very limited calories. Don't forget about this fundamental common denominator among diets. It is the singular cause of ultimate failure for dieters. Well, you might ask, how can a person possibly lose weight without forcing the restriction of calories, cutting back and controlling portions?

There is a way. It is about the principles of physiology that have kept the human race going for millennia.

Are you ready? Here we go!

# PART I

Information About Your Body That You Would Never Guess in a Million Years

# CHAPTER 1

## The Secret Life of Fat

Overweight people—you might be one of them—have too much fat on their bodies. This statement may seem rather obvious, if not absurd. But, there is a mystery about this fact, an ironic mystery, which is hidden within the ingenious bodies of the overweight. The unfolding of this mystery fills the pages of this book. No, it is not a new potion or snake oil or quick fix. It's mysterious and wonderful information about your body and why working against it never works—and how cooperating with it will lead to the change you want.

First, let's take a look at some typical stories of people who have struggled unsuccessfully over years, trying to lose this mysterious fat. *All the names and some details of the stories in this book are changed to protect their privacy.* These histories reflect the conundrum dieters everywhere are in; even when they can lose weight, they can't keep it off indefinitely. Consequently, they are forced, in a way, to try dieting over and over again, in spite of the same result.

1

## Margaret

I am a 51-year-old mother of three and grandmother of four. I have been struggling with weight—I'm 5'1" and 188 pounds—for decades. I weighed 98 pounds when I got married but after my third pregnancy, in spite of strict dieting, I slowly began to gain. I have been on low-fat, low-carb, a popular group plan, diet pills and I've joined fitness clubs many times. I am almost always on one diet or another. I have a heel spur, hypertension and high cholesterol, which really concern me, but I just don't seem to be able to get my weight down and keep it off.

## Julie

I just turned thirty-three and I realize I've been fighting the same 30 pounds all my life. I started gaining weight in college and just tried to cut back on portions. That worked for a while but the pounds crept back on when I didn't stay with my plan. Eventually I bought a popular diet book and tried that. I was successful and lost 25 pounds over a few months but eventually gained that back too. I've just repeated the same story over and over again with different diets, mostly from books, at least 10 times. Now I'm struggling to just stay at 30 pounds over where I should be, and it scares me. Even going on another diet scares me. It doesn't sound like such a big deal compared to people who struggle with real obesity, but it really affects my self-esteem and confidence because I just keep failing.

## Sarah

I'm 38 and work as a bank teller. I'm single, probably because of my weight. I was always curvy in high school and started dieting when I weighed 150. (I'm 5'5"). That decision began a very long and sad chapter in my life—I've been dieting for 16 years. I'm a lousy dieter because I can never stay with it for more than a few weeks. Then when I go off a diet, my appetite goes crazy and I always gain all the weight back. I've tried juice fasting, cleansing diets, a diet that supplies the food, quick weight loss everything, meditation, hypnosis and a weekly group plan. Now I weigh 210. I carry most of my weight in my middle and that doesn't help. I'm trying to accept my size but I admit I'm always hopeful I'll find a diet that will work for me.

## Melanie

I can't remember ever not being on a diet. I was already chubby at 8 so my mother took me with her to her diet club. I don't know if I ever lost weight, but I did get hungry trying to eat that way. I just got bigger throughout high school and felt rejected by my classmates. This led to more eating and weight gain. Now, I'm 45 and weigh 175. I'm 5'2". No diet has ever worked for me. I can't stay with most of them and even when I do lose weight, I gain it back pretty fast. And I'm already having health problems from my weight. I'm pre-diabetic. I have arthritis in my knees and hips, and sleep apnea. My parents were both pretty heavy so maybe I just inherited it.

## Peggy

I'm 5'4" tall and I weigh about 200. I have diabetes and arthritis. I've tried just about every weight-loss thing out there. I'm good at losing weight and I'm good at gaining it back. In fact, I always gain it back— all of it and usually more than I lost. A friend just underwent gastric bypass and ended up with two subsequent surgeries for obstructions, pneumonia and other problems. Not for me, thanks. But I would like to know if there is anything I can do about my weight that will last. I would like to enjoy shopping for clothes again but I seriously doubt that that's ever going to happen short of a miracle.

**What's Your Story?**

You probably can relate to these stories. But what do all these ladies have in common? Yes, obviously they all struggle with their weight, but what else? They are all dieters. Well, you may say, of course they're all dieters. They should be dieting—they're fat!

But hold on a minute. Did you notice that they are all *serious, repeat dieters*? Five, six and more diets repeated over the years. Dieting and *weight gain*—keep this connection in mind as you read ahead.

**How Do Dieters Get So Stuck?**

Let's go back and start at the beginning of these diet careers. All diets begin at the same point. People notice (or imagine) that their bodies are bigger, softer and fatter than they would like them to be. This insight has been the starting point of diets for decades: Time to find a diet that will help me to eat less and guarantee that I'll lose weight! Millions have consciously chosen this remedy over generations. Apparently, those dieters who repeatedly failed at dieting did not warn a new batch about their sad experiences. Statistically, 95 percent of dieters regain all the weight they lose within two to five years. And some researchers estimate that 60 percent gain back more weight than they lose.

But dieters are simply following a definite prescription: "Overweight people need to eat less and exercise more," one well-known obesity researcher stated confidently at the beginning of his research report. "On the surface, he says, the solution to obesity is just that simple." But then, he admits, "long-term weight loss remains an elusive goal for so many, (the vast majority), even after they have spent thousands of dollars and endured endless diets, exercise regimens, and other 'cures.'" Just about everyone, including obesity researchers, believes that people who are fat simply eat too much all the time and exercise too little. If they would just stick to eating less and exercising more, they wouldn't be fat. And these ideas sure seem to make logical sense: The more you eat, the fatter you will be and the less you eat, the thinner you will be. Is this really true?

## The Reason People are Fat—It's Not Exactly What You Think

Try to let go of everything you've ever heard/read about excess fat deposits on the body. This may be a real challenge because misinformation about body fat runs rampant. We learn that anybody with extra fat has a defective body, that extra body fat is simply evil. We certainly believe that fat has no positive function and simply must be starved/worked/walked off. And, we believe that there is absolutely no redeeming quality to excess fat on a body. So, we'd better get rid of it—as fast as possible!

The hitch in this approach is that it's not true. Fat, even excess fat on a body, is important. Fat, from the perspective of its original role in the body, is a good thing. I'm not joking.

There are reasons, very real reasons—good reasons—that fat is there, on your abdomen, thighs, arms, neck—everywhere extra padding will fit. This information may help you feel a little better about yourself. Here are the things that fat does for your body that you've probably never heard about:

Body Fat

1. cushions organs
2. provides thermal insulation
3. transports soluble vitamins
4. provides energy reserves when the food supply is inadequate

5

Pay attention to that last one: *Fat provides energy reserves when the food supply is inadequate.*

Perhaps the most important role that fat has played in the history of the human race is providing fuel for bodies during times of famine. This was tantamount to the continuation of the human species. If, during times of plenty, humans did not have the ability to store energy in the form of fat, many, most, or all would have died of starvation. Famines usually fluctuated with the seasons. Body fat storage developed as a necessary physiological adjustment from the earliest times of man. Without this adaptive potential, human beings would probably have vanished from the face of the earth.

It wasn't that long ago that there were real shifts in the availability of food even in our country, particularly for people in colder climates. Bodies in these environments experienced famines typically in the winter and early spring when the food supply was low. As summer moved into fall and food became plentiful, people prepared for famine times by extra eating during these seasons of plenty. Naturally, people stored extra food both externally and internally during abundant seasons for future use during famines.

Let's get back to a popular belief among obesity researchers, one who writes: "These ideas about survival fat only apply to our distant ancestors, or more recently, nomadic tribes who experienced harsh winters. We have plenty of food in America for everybody now, all the time. In fact, it's too much food and too much of the wrong kind of food—that's what makes people fat. It's as simple as that; fat people eat too much! They have to learn to eat less and work out, period!"

This good doctor's opinion may reflect your own attitude: There's sure plenty of food around me. In fact, you may say, I never go hungry! I'm FAT! I do eat TOO MUCH!"

Keep reading.

## Our Bodies Haven't Changed that Much

Unlike the dinosaurs, we did survive, and fat has played this crucial role in our survival. Our bodies still have a physiological sensitivity to an inadequate food supply. Just like the cavemen, we still possess the innate ability to eat in excess of current needs in order to store fuel for use later when food sources dwindle. Limited food is called a *famine* and can range from mild to severe. The survival mechanisms for bodies adjusting to famines seems antiquated to us because it looks like we always have plenty of food now, right? Food is everywhere in America today. Grocery stores exist every few miles or even every few blocks. So what's all this about an inadequate food and survival?

Health promoter Jane Brody agrees that, historically, bodies stored extra calories in the form of fat for use when the food supply became uncertain. But then she goes on to say that the food supply in 20th-century America is "hardly uncertain." And, judging from the grocery store shelves, she is right. But, dieters don't eat freely from the grocery store shelves!

You can *live* in a grocery store, but if you don't eat enough food for your body's needs, for whatever reason, your body experiences a type of famine. The fact that food is actually available, by itself, has no bearing on your body's survival responses. Your body only knows what you eat. People may have a refrigerator and cupboards full of food, but it doesn't make any difference to their bodies if they're not eating enough. Today, even in America, the food supply of every dieter, while dieting, is uncertain. And that uncertainty means the food supply is inadequate at times and the body needs energy reserves. What exactly are energy reserves?

## Fat is the Energy Reserve on a Human Body

Intermittently, dieters eat less food than they need, and because this is a famine to their bodies, this under eating triggers a protective response in their bodies—one that stimulates the need for *more* energy reserves. They actually develop a need for more energy backup fat than non-dieters. The very act of dieting causes dieters' bodies to plump up their energy reserves to get ready for the next diet. Isn't this absolutely crazy? It's the way dieters try to lose weight that makes them gain it back. Let me say that again: Eat-less dieting causes the rebound that dieters almost inevitably experience. Diets make lasting weight loss impossible.

Fat is what dieters want to lose, but they don't understand what they're doing to their bodies. When they diet, they force their bodies to quickly burn fat and *at the same time* create an increased need for fat for the future. This is why dieters always go off their diets—for the *necessary* restoration of the fat they've lost during the diet. Ironic, isn't it? And what's the evidence for this idea? Rebound statistics. Rebounding is a simply a physiological survival response. Since all dieters eventually go off their diets because of this survival mechanism, the duration of the diet or low food supply is limited and bodies get a chance to recover. And they do recover. This recovery is, for the dieter, the saddest, most frustrating and maddening time. It's the gain-it-all-back period. And, naturally, there is always a next famine—a new diet attempt to get rid of those pesky energy reserves. So the cycle goes.

## Desperate to be Thin

As a teen, there was nothing I wanted more than to be thin, and I had proved it by trying just about every diet I could find. But, I always ended up feeling out of control when I got to a certain point in a diet. Other dieters confided that they experienced this, too. I knew it was not an excuse, it really happened. I was highly motivated. I was educated. I was an R.N. for crying out loud. If anyone should be able to diet successfully, it was I. But no matter how hard I tried, I could not keep from overeating at some point in my dieting efforts. Eventually, I always became exhausted, frustrated, confused and overweight.

At my crisis point, 17 years into dieting, I began to search for a real solution to my weight and dieting problems. Actually, my dieting lifestyle was as big a problem as my weight by this time. My obsession with my weight leaked into every aspect of my life. It made me depressed, it made me anxious, it ruined my self-esteem and preoccupied my thoughts. When I was dieting "successfully" I was constantly fighting my hunger and when I was gaining the weight back I was constantly berating myself for my lack of willpower. I was obsessed. I was almost possessed! I kept asking this same question: Why was I overeating?

## Looking For Answers in Other Places

I had learned about the principles of adaptation in nurse's training and began to look at obesity and dieting from the perspective of survival. As I connected the dots about the role of fat in survival, a light went on, and then another light. Gradually, I began to see fat as some kind of survival tool, and that certain physical needs—like food—somehow triggered it. Once I figured out that dieting—under eating—was connected to my overeating, my overeating began to make sense. My attitude toward my body changed and I became hopeful. I realized then, that I had to actually stop dieting and cooperate with my body's survival needs if I was ever going to get off the yo-yo diet cycle and lose weight for good. Stop dieting? Whoa Nelly!

## About Face

I had figured out that my dieting actually set me up to overeat and to regain weight. I was powerless to lose weight and keep it off as long as I kept dieting the way I did. I realized that I had to *learn to eat*. Now this was a switch! The very thing I had feared—food—had become the key to my lasting weight loss. No wonder I had been stuck in a no-win lifestyle for so long. My weight loss tactics were physiologically programmed to backfire. My willpower wasn't the problem, except that it was focused in the wrong direction. I had plenty of willpower, but I had to learn to use it differently if I ever wanted to conquer my struggles with my body.

It may still seem totally counterintuitive that eating *less* can eventually lead to weight *gain*, but look at your own diet history and you will see a pattern. Even though you may have lost a lot of weight over the years, have you ever been able to keep it off? Why have you given up on a successful diet even though you felt better, looked better, and your whole life was better when you were thin? Have you gradually grown heavier? Are you less and less able to tolerate diets or lose any weight when you try?

As I thought of obesity from this new survival perspective, pieces of the common yo-yo diet experience began to make sense. I realized that fat bodies are doing what they are programmed to do. Over time and because of my own experience, I became confident that excess fat on bodies subjected to dieting is a positive adaptation where the food supply is sometimes limited. We suffer other problems from being overweight, but those problems are clearly not as important as survival.

As I read research articles and books on diet and weight loss, it became apparent that no one was looking at the typical American weight-loss diet from the body's perspective—as a threat. In fact, everyone seemed to believe that dieting and going hungry are normal, healthy behaviors.

## Adrienne

Adrienne's experience with a popular medically supervised rapid weight loss diet illustrates this principle. This diet is a severely food restricted program for rapid weight loss for obese people. A 28-year old librarian, Adrienne was supervised by nurses and a physician because of the risks of very rapid weight loss, but the rapid weight loss was exactly why she was there. She'd been on just about every eat-less/exercise-more program and she was sick of gaining back weight she'd worked so hard to lose. She was desperate to shed the 95 pounds she'd gained over the past 15 years.

As promised, Adrienne lost weight very fast, so fast that her skin hung on her after she'd shed 50 pounds—a little over 4 months into her diet. She was so encouraged, she threw her "fat" clothes in the garbage and bought new ones, even smaller than she had become. Adrienne was confident she'd reach her goal, and the medical staff was, too. She was not disappointed.

Then, Adrienne went on the maintenance program, which offered more food options and slightly larger portions. It was clearly better than the mostly liquid diet she'd been on for several months. She had strict guidelines for what to eat and how much in order to keep her weight down. There was some flexibility but she knew she had to stick with the restrictions for good or she'd throw it all away again. She got a lot of support from her team and her family. She looked like a different person. She felt like a different person. The compliments were effusive and people were genuinely impressed.

About six months after she attained her goal weight, Adrienne found herself hungrier than she'd been and thinking about foods she knew were off her list. When she weighed herself, she was up six pounds. She panicked and made an appointment with her nurse. Back on track for a while, Adrienne again experienced almost overpowering hunger and strong cravings. These led to occasional bingeing and a preference for sweets.

It took Adrienne only two years to regain the 95 pounds she'd lost.

## The Half Plate Diet

A veteran dieter of 22 years, Janet knew overeating was her problem. She had 55 extra pounds to prove it. She said she just couldn't keep the control she needed to get to her goal weight. Sometime during every diet she'd end up eating too much and all the wrong kinds of food. So, at one point, she began to design her own diets, thinking that maybe the diets were at fault for the weight rebounds she experienced. The most recent diet Janet made up was simple; she'd just eat half of anything on her plate. She thought the deprivation of most of her diets had set her up to fail, so, she didn't deprive herself of any type of food and said she enjoyed eating and never missed a meal. This sounds like a perfectly sane approach on the surface, and Janet lost nearly 50 pounds over a year. She was encouraged and thought she'd finally found the answer. Unfortunately, she gradually gained 60 pounds over the following two years. Janet had found a track that worked for her but it didn't work for her body.

Because it is logical that too much food causes obesity, we have been preoccupied with the overeating part of the equation. It is true that some people really do just eat too much, including too much calorie-dense food, and that certainly contributes to, and possibly causes, their weight problems, but we're not talking about them. We are talking about dieters who go hungry on purpose to lose weight. We have ignored the part that sparks the overeating—the under eating. Overeating looks like such an obvious culprit, and the idea that dieting—eating less—could be the problem in your weight loss efforts may still seem preposterous.

If it were really so simple to lose weight by dieting, dieters everywhere would be blissfully thin and able to stick with their eat-less/do-more programs. We know that's not true. In fact, many dieters are a lot fatter than they were when they started dieting. If the popular diet approach was really effective, would we be so fat and so stuck after 60 years of doing it?

## Two Questions Never Objectively Explored

Two questions have never been *objectively* asked by obesity specialists: First, if overeating causes obesity, what really causes overeating? And second, why do overweight people prefer to overeat particularly bad foods?

The reason obesity specialists never seriously ask these questions is because they think they already know the answers: Of course, they say, people overeat because they love to eat and they love to eat fattening foods because they taste good and they just don't care and they don't have any self-control and they are emotionally stunted and so they eat so much they get addicted and then they can't stop so they get fatter and fatter and fatter! It's as if there's no mystery to this question at all: The cause of overeating and choosing lousy food is self-indulgence and emotional struggles that go out of control. People eat too much because they are psychologically sick and food addicts! Right? Well.

Perhaps some of these explanations have some truth to them, but they are overly simplistic. Many highly educated obesity researchers, physicians, trainers, nurses, and other health professionals, overeat at times and eat foods they know they shouldn't. So, it isn't so simple. There's more going on than emotional issues and food lust. We know this because many people are thin and living in the very same food environment as the overweight, with heavy emotions and food all around them.

These theories about why people overeat and prefer lousy food are popular among the overweight and obese too. Let's look at one specific theory that we all have been taught explains overeating: People overeat because of their emotions. This is an almost universally accepted idea, but I never bought into the notion that emotions are to blame for overeating. It is a convenient thing to blame for otherwise inexplicable behaviors.

## Food for Feelings?

Research simply does not support the idea that overeating is emotionally driven. Studies have shown, despite discrimination in both academic and work settings; overweight people show no greater psychological disturbance than non-obese people. Overweight people do face struggles and emotional problems because they are human and, perhaps partly, because they are fat in a culture that rejects fat people. So this research debunks the idea that overweight people are emotional jellyfish who deal with their psychological problems by eating. The idea that people overeat simply because of their emotions is terribly depressing because all people are emotional. The good news, if you have thought of yourself as an emotional overeater, is that you'll soon learn that this "diagnosis" doesn't apply to you in the way you have thought. You can be forever freed from the scourge of "emotional eating."

Every human being is emotional but not everyone is overweight. Therefore, many people who feel stressed, fearful, worried, upset, nervous, anxious, terrified, intimidated, sad, hurt, disappointed, ashamed, confused, resentful, frustrated, guilty, embarrassed, angry, or disturbed, do not eat in response to these feelings. There's a logical reason for this fact and it's not because they have more fortitude than emotional overeaters. The reason some overeating is blamed on emotions is because bingeing and emotions show up together. There's a real explanation for this coincidence, but it's not cause/effect. I'll explain this connection in Chapter 6, dedicated to the emotional overeating theory, as well as the food addiction idea and the use of behaviorism as a tool for weight loss.

Why do overweight people so often eat particularly poor quality food? Although taste preference and habit may play very significant roles, there is something else less apparent happening in many over weights who eat lousy food. Whenever anybody becomes overly hungry on a regular basis, whether from dieting or just reckless eating patterns, they are likely to be more interested in foods that are fat producing. This too is a physiological phenomenon, and will be discussed in the next chapter, Why Dieting Backfires.

## How People Gain Weight in the First Place

Dieting isn't the only way to experience a famine, although it's a particularly obvious and concerted one. People everywhere experience some kind of food restriction and/or eat very poor quality food. Just like going hungry regularly, eating a lot of poor quality food triggers the body's survival response. Lousy food doesn't satisfy the body's need for nutrients. There are several ways to under eat besides dieting. One of the big reasons the obesity rate is skyrocketing is that people fall into these common habits. These habits mimic those of dieters because they involve under eating on some level. People go hungry even though they are not dieting: They miss meals because they are in a hurry. They don't take time to prepare and eat meals or snacks. Most people don't take food with them for times when food is inaccessible. They don't recognize the symptoms of hunger, and consequently, don't eat when they need to. Job schedules often interfere with workers' ability to eat meals or snacks when they are hungry. Poor quality food is regular fare for many people and families at home, school, and work. And, it is common for people to ignore their hunger because eating is inconvenient and they don't realize how important it is to avoid going hungry.

Very often, the unconscious habit of going hungry during the day and then overeating at night is a daily pattern. Sometimes it is weekly, with overeating on the weekend. These patterns lead to weight gain and maintenance of excess weight in most people.

## Thomas

A hospital orderly, 33-year old Thomas has a physically demanding job. He is at work by 7:00 a.m. He has a long rush hour commute each morning so he doesn't have time for breakfast. Coffee is available on each unit when he gets to work and that's all he has until his lunch break at 1:30 PM. Thomas often misses lunch because he is busy, which doesn't bother him because he figures he needs to lose weight anyway. If he has time, he goes to the cafeteria with a co-worker for lunch, but the fare isn't very appetizing to him. He usually has two yogurts and a Coke, maybe some French fries. At break time, Thomas slips out to the vending machines for candy bars, even though he knows they aren't good for him. By this time he's aware that he is very hungry. Typically, Thomas stops on the way home after work at a fast food restaurant and orders two double cheeseburgers, a large fries with a large soda. Still hungry later, Thomas cooks a frozen pizza, and has chips and dip and beer as he watches TV. Ice cream is always ready in the freezer. Thomas is 70 pounds overweight.

This is a pattern so common that it universally promotes weight gain in even the most dedicated gym member. It's easier to go hungry earlier in the day: You are well rested. Your work environment is more stimulating than the lunchroom and not as conducive to eating as evening at home. It's just easier to drink pop, coffee or water and pass up the lunch and snacks—breakfast too. Hunger in this pattern is usually mild until mid afternoon and then it tends to become more demanding. By the time you get to dinner, you are famished and needing big or second helpings.

## More About Eating Patterns

When overweight people aren't actually dieting, many try to avoid food, even subconsciously. Like Thomas, they usually skip breakfast because they are still full from overeating the night before, or they are simply not hungry, or they can tolerate hunger better when they are not tired, or they want to skip the calories, or they don't have time to eat. They might skip lunch too, or eat something light, especially if they are with other people. For many overweight and obese people, eating in front of other people is uncomfortable. They may feel as if they don't deserve to be eating food, in light of how fat they are.

In the rebound phase, overweight people indulge their appetites and cravings, in private and/or in public. If they eat in public, this is the time when their reputation for overeating is observed and often quietly judged. Research has shown that overweight people, on the whole, eat less than people of normal weight. But this is not true during the rebound phase. Overeating and choosing rich, fat-producing foods are the hallmarks of any dieter in rebound.

## Eating Too Much

We've established that typically people eat too much and all the wrong stuff because they aren't eating enough of the right stuff—at the right time. They experience famines from which they must recover. The food supply in America today is both fantastic and frighteningly poor, even disgusting. Many non-foods, meaning foods that are almost completely artificial and devoid of nutrients, are available. These foods are often calorie-dense and fattening, even when they are labeled low fat, sugar-free and "diet." But our quality food supply is also amazingly varied and plentiful throughout the year! In light of famine and feast idea, it is not so great a mystery why millions of Americans are choosing the former over the latter.

Our bodies still possess the adaptive potential to take in more food, qualitatively and quantitatively, than we need to live. Naturally, this is easy to do given a plethora of sugary, salty, fatty, low-class, poor-nutrient, excessively portioned, tasty, habit-forming fake foods. It seems that a full quarter of the grocery store shelves are stocked with these items and many shoppers consider them staples. They are not.

Do people get fat just eating these foods regularly? Definitely. Calorie-rich "pleasure" foods contribute significantly to obesity, even cause it in some people. But I have found that many of those people who indulge in foods like this also eat erratically, missing meals, and going hungry at times. So, they experience both quantity famines—not enough food at the right time—and quality famines—not enough good food.

## How does a body do it?

Dieters' bodies use several specific and ingenious means to adjust to the low-fuel threat that a typical diet brings. A discussion about these amazing body responses is coming up in Chapter 2. Bodies are built to adapt to environmental changes, not to comply with psychological needs and goals. Dieters' bodies must work hard to protect them from themselves, or they would surely starve themselves to death. Instead, with the exception of anorexics, who really may be in danger of death, most of us have bodies that demonstrate their capacity to survive dieting by adding pounds.

Just remember this fact: When fat becomes a survival priority to a body in famine off and on, the body adopts amazing physiological adjustments to ensure survival. These adjustments or adaptations are specific and universal. Now you know *why* bodies change in these ways, and that's cleared up some confusion. But now it's time to learn about exactly *what*'s going on and *how* it all works.

Get ready to explore how dieters' bodies work behind the scenes. These are probably some of the most mysterious physiological phenomena of adaptation, and probably the most misinterpreted. For example, loss of control over eating (bingeing) has been almost universally considered psychological or emotional. It is not. Learn how even bingeing fits into the logic of survival. It is one powerful example of the body's ability to influence eating behavior in order to survive. This "feasting" that follows a diet famine is the central topic in the next chapter. It is crucial to understanding how the body fights for survival against the struggling dieter. But feasting isn't the whole picture. There's a lot more going on. Get ready for more AHA experiences!

# CHAPTER 2

## Why Dieting Backfires

Rebound weight gain in dieters is so common that it has become an adage. We witness the weight-loss rebound all around us—in movie stars, diet spokespersons, our neighbors, ourselves. And, we speculate: Is *loss of willpower* to blame? Is it just *falling back into old eating patterns*? Is it apathy—do dieters just *not care enough* to keep it off?

Well, it's more complicated than that, as you know by now. Diet rebound is not just a function of overeating, emotions or lost willpower, even though we have thought this way for decades. Remember, the underlying truth is in the principles of adaptation and survival. The rebound phenomenon is about bodies surviving diet famines by prompting necessary feasts. The principles of adaptation and survival offer compelling explanations for these maddening realities. And, these explanations challenge, and even contradict, the typical diet regimen in this country. At the same time, they provoke other questions that must be answered: Exactly *how* do bodies fight against dieters' eat-less efforts, and *how* do dieters gain back the weight they lose?

## Exactly How Bodies Sabotage Dieters

There are five specific ways that bodies react to dieting, fighting dieters' efforts to lose weight and, ultimately, causing dieters to fail. These five adaptations to dieting (famine) can be divided into two categories: *energy conservation* and *preventing weight loss.*

### Energy conservation:

### *Bodies protect fuel reserves by*

1. *Lowering the metabolic rate*
2. *Lowering energy and activity levels*

Let's look at the first way bodies fight dieters:

### *Bodies protect fuel reserves by lowering the metabolic rate.*

Many dieters complain that this "problem" applies to them. It does! Dieters really do experience lowered metabolic rate when they restrict their eating. This decrease in metabolism is simply an adaptation to the decreased food intake. In order to continue functioning on a limited fuel supply, a body must lower its basic fuel needs. So, a body in famine adjusts to getting along on the restricted fuel intake. Oxygen consumption goes down and the core body temperature drops. These are a few of the obvious changes the body goes through. The problem with this energy conserving change is that these fuel efficiency tactics may continue beyond the end of the diet, even after food is plentiful.

Marian Apfelbaum, M.D. was involved in hundreds of research studies on obesity and weight loss. His research showed that the metabolic rate of people who are dieting drops by 15 percent to 30 percent. This is why dieters often complain of feeling tired, apathetic and unmotivated.

George Bray M.D. discovered a 20 percent decrease in metabolic rate in as little as two weeks of dieting—a decrease measurable within 48 hours of caloric restriction. This big decrease in baseline energy expenditure suggests the bodies become even more metabolically efficient, lowering energy use because food restriction from any source, external or internal, signals danger to the body, he said.

A number of obesity researchers (Boyle, Storlien and Keesey, and others) showed that repeated calorie restriction in animals might have *permanent effects* on metabolism. The researchers interpreted the findings to mean that that these metabolic depressions were adaptations to food restriction. So, simply put, bodies react fast to under eating by lowering energy expenditure, and over time repeated food restriction may cause a lasting depression of metabolic rate. This implies that there is a possibility that, with long-term dieting, individuals may actually make it more and more difficult to lose weight at all. I have heard such testimonies.

**The Best of Intentions**

When metabolism is depressed, dieters' bodies reflect this:

### *Bodies protect fuel reserves by lowering energy and activity levels.*

Underfed bodies are likely to be more tired and less inclined to move around unnecessarily. This is easy to understand if you think about a real famine. Let's say you get lost in a forest without any food for several days. During that time, your body adjusts to the lack of food by conserving surface heat. You get cold, literally. And you want to sit down. You may even get sleepy.

Among dieters, those who drop out of an exercise program are the rule rather than the exception. In a 1980 study, researchers Kelly Brownell, PhD, and Albert Stunkard, M.D., found that 50 percent of overweight people who were prescribed a weight-loss exercise program drop out, even when they had "compelling medical reasons" to adhere to it. Many other researchers confirmed this finding.

## Roy

Roy's story is about his body's protection of fuel reserves by avoidance of physical activity. Roy suffered a heart attack. His doctor put him on a low-calorie, low-fat and low-salt diet. In addition, the doctor prescribed a workout regimen.

After two weeks, Roy quit the workouts, although he tried to stay with the diet. He quit exercising in spite of the advice of his doctor, who said, "If you don't exercise, you could die." When he quit going to the gym, he told his wife, "If I *do* keep exercising, I probably *will* die!" Roy's body won over his doctor's advice—he wasn't able to keep the work out regimen going on so little fuel.

The drop in metabolic rate and the reluctance to move around are related. When the metabolism drops, energy drops, too. This might be subtle but its influence is always significant. People with hypothyroidism, whose metabolisms are below normal, experience a common symptom—fatigue. It makes sense that tired people are less likely to be active. So it is with dieters.

Perhaps the dieter doesn't notice the impact of the diet on her metabolism. She just joined a club and enlisted a trainer, so how can you say that she's avoiding physical activity? It's possible to trump the body's adaptive responses—for a while. This is why dieters tend to stop and start their workouts. But, keep in mind that there is a battle going on between dieters and their bodies. Unfortunately for dieters, they are unlikely to win in the long run. The statistics are woefully against them.

**The Battle:**

*Bodies protect fuel reserves by fighting weight loss and preparing to regain by*

1. *Increased appetite*
2. *Cravings for sweet and fatty food*
3. *Preoccupation with food and eating*

### *Bodies resist weight loss by increasing the appetite.*

Obesity researcher Aaron Altschul said, "Your body doesn't know you're dieting. It thinks you're starving, and in response mobilizes every hormone, every brain chemical, every mood, any craving it can manipulate to make you restore the lost weight. As a result, many dieters gain back all the weight they lost, plus a little more."

Most dieters will readily admit that their appetites tend to increase and, sometimes soar when they start a new eat-less plan. But, not all dieters experience this, at least not at first. Some swear that they are "never hungry" and that the food limits don't pose a problem for them. This is another great example of the adaptive potential of the human body. Some don't experience extra hunger in spite of the deprivation because their bodies are adjusting to the limited food supply. These bodies take the logical route, as if to say, Why send hunger signals when this is all we're going to get anyway? So the dieters may not feel hungrier—yet. But, there comes a day in all dieters' lives when the hunger catches up with them. Sometimes, it is all of a sudden, and sometimes, it just creeps up. When it does, the diet goes to waste.

It's obvious that increased appetite combats dieters' efforts to lose weight by self-imposed famines. Increased appetite, often experienced after a period of "good dieting," may lead to overeating or bingeing. This is why some diets include "cheat" days. Dieters *need* to have a day or two off to catch up on their eating. Sooner or later, the body accomplishes efficient fat storage, in part, by an increased appetite. This is an important part of the battle, and you know who's going to win.

### Bodies resist weight loss by shifting cravings to fat-producing foods.

Dieters eventually experience this phenomenon when they embark on a food-restricted diet: Their cravings shift to sweeter, higher fat foods. Dieters don't, as a rule, crave broccoli. Why?

Remember that bodies in famine adapt to the low availability of food. This creates a biological need to store fat *when possible*. So, bodies get the signal from food restriction to eat more food that is calorie-condensed, in an attempt to increase overall fuel intake. Besides an increase in appetite, dieters usually crave foods made from concentrated mixtures of sugar and fat—excellent fat producers, perfect for bodies recovering from famines. Vegetables and fruits aren't especially calorie rich and consequently not good fat producers. So, dieters don't fantasize about broccoli. They don't *need* broccoli. They *need* fat, so naturally, they crave foods like chocolate and ice cream.

The director of human nutrition at a major university, Adam Drenowski, found that yo-yo dieting creates cravings for a calorie-dense mixture of sugar and fat. Now we know *why* this shift in cravings goes in the direction of fat-producers.

## Bodies resist weight loss by preoccupation with food.

The third biological adaptation to dieting may be subtle, but not so mysterious when you think about it. Preoccupation with food and eating sounds like a psychological phenomenon, doesn't it? It sure does, but it isn't. Research with *food-restricted normal-weight volunteers* showed that they experienced significant preoccupation with food, as well as many of the other symptoms that dieters experience. Threats to survival put the body on high alert. If food intake is maintained below survival levels, as it is in a typical weight-loss diet, the body quickly focuses on food and eating.

This adaptive response is frustrating to dieters who are on a limited food regimen. They strive to distract themselves from it and do so by many means. They work out because intense physical exercise can depress the appetite. They drink—coffee, tea, sodas, water, shakes, smoothies and energy drinks. Sometimes, they drink alcoholic beverages. They prefer drinks that do not contain calories because calories are the enemy. Unfortunately for them, no-calorie drinks, especially the ones with caffeine, often leave dieters weak and nervous. Shakes and smoothies are better because they contain calories, but they often serve as substitutes for meals. The trouble there is that liquid "meals" do not last very long in keeping hunger at bay, especially with exercise. So, hunger and preoccupation with food typically return within a short time.

**Here's a review of how bodies fight dieters:**

1. Drop in metabolic rate—15-30%
2. Low energy and reluctance for physical activity
3. Increased appetite
4. Cravings for sweets and fatty foods
5. Preoccupation with food and eating

So when dieters go on an eat-less, exercise-more diet, they unknowingly trigger their bodies to adapt in these five ways. Taken together, these five adaptations protect the fat already there and may eventually promote even more fat accumulation. *These changes do not seem to occur at first, of course.* The rewarding weight loss comes first. But these adaptations, transmitted by biochemical changes, lie in wait, eventually causing the dieter to lose control of her eating. And when they take over, the frustration and weight gain begin.

Remember, bodies cannot distinguish between famines that are "real" and famines that are self-imposed. Bodies don't know that food isn't available because of an accident or the season, or because you weighed yourself that morning and vowed to eat only celery and apples. Accidental famines happen to everyone. We all get stuck in situations where we get hungry and there is no food. (Solving this problem is crucial to recovery and will be addressed later.) But the vast majority of famines happen because we deeply believe that too much food, by itself, makes us fat.

**Who Knew?**

Dieters wage a personal war against their bodies that they can't possibly win. But they do stay valiantly in control of their eating—their portions, their menu, and their mealtimes—for a while. This shows that pure will and determination can overcome the body's survival mechanisms, right? Yes, but this temporary part of the war is really just a skirmish. Some times it's a month, sometimes three or six months or even a year that they are able to stay with a restrictive diet program. It's admirable. Often they lose a significant amount of weight during this time, and experience all the perks of their new body. But there comes a time when they can't go on under eating. They lose control, either suddenly or gradually. Usually the experience is confusing at best. The idea that they've actually lost control of their food intake does not occur to them. They blame themselves, they blame the sprained ankle, they blame their ex-boyfriend. But the five ways their bodies are programmed to fight them for control of food intake is the real reason they lose their grip.

**You've Got to be Kidding**

Here's a sad and ironic fact: During diets, our bodies use fuel sources within to make up for external food shortages. Calorie-deprived bodies use two main internal sources for energy: fat and lean muscle tissue. Fat is relatively light and bulky. It takes up a lot of space but doesn't actually weigh as much as muscle, which makes it an especially efficient energy storage system. Muscle on the other hand, is dense and heavy. The first type of fuel source used by the body in a famine is muscle tissue. The reason bodies use muscle for emergency fuel is this: After using up glycogen, which is stored in the liver, bodies burn muscle for fuel if the demand is immediate rather than gradual. Bodies also burn fat to keep fueled during famines, as a more gradual fuel source. It is estimated that 25 percent of weight lost by traditional dieting is *muscle tissue*, depending on the speed of weight loss and amount of exercise, and about 75 percent is fat.

The equation above is significant because it affects body composition after a diet is over. When dieters stop dieting and gain lost weight back, they don't gain the same amount of lean muscle tissue they've lost, they gain nearly *all fat*. So the diet cycle of weight loss/weight gain leads to an overall *increase in percentage of body fat*. Why does this happen? We know that bodies intermittently experiencing famine generally need more fat, right? They need more fat even *more than* muscle. We also know that the body gets what it needs most *in the recovery period.* There you have it.

## Voila!

Is this why we are so fat when we are the most diet-conscious nation on earth? It has a lot to do with it. The connection between our diet-obsessed country and our obesity statistics is undeniable when you consider the overall effect of quick weight loss dieting on the body. We have been approaching the weight problem from a completely wrong direction for over fifty years, and it shows. The terrible truth about dieting is that, for most people, not only does it fail in solving weight problems; it actually *causes weight gain* for most dieters over the long run.

Does dieting singularly cause weight problems and obesity? No, definitely not. Reckless eating habits, dangerously poor food, lack of education regarding diet and food (both the public and medical professionals), rampant advertising of poor quality food, fast food control of school menus, and particularly advertising for quick weight loss diets and "diet" foods.

## Mary

Mary's first famine happened when she was 14. She decided she was fat, even though her mother told her she was not fat. When she started going to a diet center, her mother said, "Well, it won't hurt you. Maybe it will keep you from getting fat like me." Neither Mary nor her mother knew where this decision would eventually lead.

In spite of the fact that Mary was at her ideal weight, her weight loss goal was 15 pounds. Mary was fine with that. So on her new program,

Mary lost weight, and she felt good about it! Naturally, weight loss in overweight people, or those who think they are overweight, is very encouraging. There is a sense of pride, accomplishment, control, even euphoria when people trying to lose weight actually manage to do it. For Mary, it looked like this group support program would work for her. She was so excited, and got a lot of compliments from friends. Her total weight loss was 10 pounds.

But after four or five months on the diet, Mary started eating more than her diet allowance. She knew she was cheating but she just felt so hungry! Gradually she fell off her diet and began to gain. Mary hadn't factored in this extra hunger. She felt she couldn't help but cheat on her eating program. Her appetite became more and more demanding! As she overate and gained weight, she blamed herself and felt like a failure. She felt embarrassed and ashamed of her lack of control.

Mary lived with her discouragement while her weight crept up. As she fought with her appetite and cravings, she ended up gaining 13 pounds— the 10 that she had lost and three more. Once the rebound phase was complete and Mary's weight leveled off, something remarkable happened to Mary's thinking. This change is the phenomenon that leads to the continuation of the yo-yo diet cycle. It's called "denial." After she spent time away from the pain of both dieting and rebounding, Mary developed a new determination to lose weight again. And so, she adopted a plan that was advertised on TV, which guaranteed a 10-pound weight loss in two weeks. Mary resumed control for her eating and started her new diet, excited that she could reverse most of the damage in two short weeks. Mary was on her way to 23 years of dieting that ultimately contributed to her gaining nearly 100 pounds.

## The Feast or Famine Cycle

They say that a picture is worth a thousand words. I believe it's true, and certainly applies to the illustration of the diet cycle. What follows is a picture of what millions of unfortunate dieters experience much of the time. This cycle is truly vicious, causing pain, frustration, shame and confusion. Dieters on this cycle can end up feeling crazy.

Begin with FAMINE at the top and move clockwise.

The feast or famine cycle usually starts with a famine, a diet, or other food restriction.

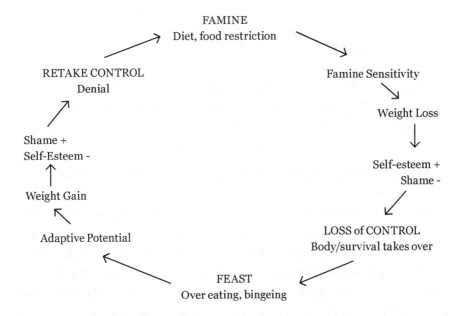

FAMINE
Diet, food restriction

RETAKE CONTROL
Denial

Famine Sensitivity

Weight Loss

Shame +
Self-Esteem -

Self-esteem +
Shame -

Weight Gain

Adaptive Potential

LOSS of CONTROL
Body/survival takes over

FEAST
Over eating, bingeing

**FAMINE**

Remember, this pattern usually begins with a Famine—you are determined to lose weight by controlling your eating, limiting portions, cutting back on calories or fat grams, or carbohydrates—whatever. Any method of under eating will set the cycle in motion, even accidental under eating for people who are susceptible. Famines are the stimulus for everything that follows:

1. Lowered metabolic rate
2. Decreased activity level
3. Increased appetite
4. Cravings for sweets and fats,
5. Preoccupation with food

**FAMINE SENSITIVITY**

Famine Sensitivity is the biological sensitivity to food restriction. The severity of the diet is a big factor and includes how restricted your eating is as well as the intensity of your activity level.

**IMPROVED SELF-ESTEEM and DIMINISHED SHAME**

As we have noted, weight loss is a wonderful thing to dieters, *the* most wonderful thing! They spend a lot of time, energy and money on this goal. And there are real psychological benefits of weight loss. Overweight people may feel badly about their bodies and their failure as dieters. When they lose weight, they get a boost in self-esteem and shake off some of their shame. They are finally *doing it!*

And as they shed the pounds, these positive emotional effects help reinforce their efforts. Weight loss gives dieters confidence and hope that their lives can really be different. These reinforcements keeps them dieting in spite of the discomfort, the inconvenience, the money, and all the stresses that go with battling their bodies.

## LOSS OF CONTROL

I have never heard of any diet program that mentioned what to do about losing control of your eating. The loss of control over eating that dieters experience is the single most important factor responsible for dieters' rebound. Rebound may happen at any time during the weight loss or maintenance. Remember, when dieters go out of control their cravings go straight to foods that will efficiently store fat because fat is what their bodies need.

The reason diet programs don't talk about the loss-of-control phenomenon is because they are only in the *weight loss business*. Staying in control during the diet and maintaining the weight loss is your problem. Have you ever thought about why the TV diet commercials are all about "I *lost* so many pounds?" I lost 50 pounds. I lost 85 pounds. I lost 66 pounds. No one talks about how long they've been able to stay there. Once in a while you'll hear someone say "And I kept it off!" Really? For three months? Or six months? It doesn't mean anything.

When I was a freshman in college, I lost about 30 pounds by starving myself spring semester. I looked great. I felt good, too. Right after that diet success, we went to California, to the beach, for a family reunion. It was fun, running around on the sandy streets, eating chocolate-covered bananas. Everything was fine right up to dinnertime the first night. We had pork chops prepared with apples. I ate fifteen of them. I became so sick that my mother almost took me to the ER. If a psychologist had been there, I would have been instantly diagnosed as psychologically disturbed or food addicted. To tell the truth though, I just went post-diet feasting crazy. I lost control—on pork chops, of all things! But wait! Those pork chops were drenched in brown sugar and butter. That was the beginning of the end of my 30-pound weight loss. I gained it all back by the end of the summer.

## FEAST

A feast plumps up the fat reserves. When dieters begin to over eat and fall off their diets, they generally know. But they don't understand and they can't help it. Really. They may find excuses: It was that cruise, or my mother's illness, or I got sick, or I had surgery or I sprained my foot and couldn't work out. Often, there is some good reason they point to. But the truth is, they just begin the feast phase because their bodies won't put up with too little food.

So, what does a feast look like? It may start rather suddenly with binge eating: bigger portions, comfort food, sweets and high fat foods. This is obvious and pretty alarming to a dieter trying to hold on to weight loss. But a feast can be more subtle and gradual—desserts slip in more often, food quality suffers, exercise is rare. The types of foods that usually make up a feast are the classic fattening foods you never see on a weight loss diet: Ice cream, cookies, pastries, chips, candy, chocolate and fried anything—any form of concentrated calories in the form of sugar, fat, and processed carbohydrates. For example, look at the ingredients in a chocolate cake: Sugar, butter, flour, chocolate, (sugar, butter, sugar, butter, etc.). How does your body instinctively know about these ingredients? Clearly it does know, and through calculated cravings, has the power to drive you, even against your will, to eat fat producers like these. It's what a feast is all about.

**Feasting Just Isn't What It Used to Be**

Let's go back to the nomadic people in the past. When feasting followed a famine, the types and amounts of food they ate to recover from the famine were restricted to the natural environmental food supply. In other words, tribal peoples of the distant past could only feast on very limited types and amounts of food.

We have come a long way since those times. Unfortunately, the foods available to us for feasting are artificially packed with fat-producing ingredients. Now we know that when we diet we experience the same famines that the people who lived off the land did. The difference is that we have access to the most notoriously fattening foods for our famine recovery. This accounts for the degree of obesity and morbid obesity in our society. Are the sugar and fat-laden foods entirely to blame? Many believe that eliminating these potent fat-producers will solve the obesity problem. This is naïve. These foods are available to everyone and yet do not "produce" obesity in all. Even thin people eat sweets, desserts and rich foods. So, it is not the foods per se, but the role they play in dysfunctional eating patterns which make them significant contributors to weight gain. These foods interact with the feast or famine cycle to produce a perfect set up for bingeing on an epic scale.

**ADAPTIVE POTENTIAL**

Adaptive potential is the capacity of the individual to meet the present and future requirements of any stimulus situation. The stimulus we're addressing is the famine experience—an intermittent limitation in the food supply. The capacity to adapt to a restricted food supply is related to famine sensitivity but also to other physical and psychological variables.

The focus of adaptive potential may be either currently based or projected into the future. Fat accumulation in bodies exposed to famine is a positive adaptation because it prepares the body for survival during future famines. Again, this suggests that your weight problem, however painful for you, is a very good thing for your body.

## WEIGHT GAIN

This is the hardest, saddest, worst part of the diet cycle. Finally, the thing we feared the most is happening. Our clothes grow tighter. If we dare weigh ourselves we see the numbers climbing. We try to hold on and keep the eating under control. We make vows. We pretend it's just a temporary setback. We try new tactics like juicing or cutting out carbs. But sooner or later the weight comes back. Not all at once, but eventually, and we end up right here we started; fat and miserable.

## LOWER SELF-ESTEEM, MORE SHAME

I don't know anyone who isn't sensitive about gaining weight, who doesn't feel worse about her/himself when those numbers on the scale go up and the jeans get tight. Just as weight loss is affirming and encouraging, weight gain is depressing. Many people who lose the diet war feel defeated and self-rejecting, even guilty. They may feel ashamed and embarrassed when they fail at dieting. They know that people look at them and think they don't even try—but dieters do try!

## DENIAL

There is a saying that I've heard in chemical dependence centers: Denial ain't no river in Egypt. The human spirit is remarkably resilient. We resist defeat. We pick ourselves up and try all over again. We keep on keeping on. We never give up. We try different angles. We invent a different tool. We are innovative. These are good traits and account for much success in people's lives. But when it comes to dieting, this willingness to try and try the same thing again puts us in the grip of the feast or famine cycle—the never-ending weight loss, weight gain merry-go-round.

Dieting makeovers abound and we are ripe for the picking because we don't want to give up on something as important as our bodies. We slip into denial when, having regained all the weight back from the last diet—or perhaps just a portion of it—we look for a new, different, proven method to lose weight. Remembering Chapter 1, we all know what this looks like and where it leads.

## REGAIN CONTROL

Regaining control over our eating and appetite comes with the next famine—the new diet. Having come full circle, rebounding and getting settled into the higher weight, we are determined to win this time. Girded by denial and a brand new diet program with special features and promises, we embark once again, knowing we can control our wayward appetites and stick to the new, improved program forever. Once we are on our way, losing weight once again, we get that infusion of optimism and good feelings about ourselves.

## OK, IT'S TIME TO DIET!

And there it is.

## What's Happening Behind the Scenes?

Remember the five ways that bodies adjust to any famine experience that we talked about in Chapter 1? Here they are again: Lowered metabolic rate, decreased physical activity, increased appetite, and cravings for sweets and fatty foods. Don't forget, once a famine is underway, all bodies kick into this five-point preservation mode. They do this by producing bio-chemicals in response to under eating. Researchers have identified some of these bio-chemicals. More on this fascinating topic in Chapter 6.

## So Where Do We Go from Here If Dieting Always Backfires?

It doesn't make sense that you can just eat and eat and lose weight, does it? No, it doesn't. Eating less food than your body is using *is required for weight loss*, but there's a vast difference between waging war with your body and making peace instead. This entire book is filled with descriptions of the war—we know all about that. So, what does peace with your body look like? To put it simply, the famines end. The famines are the crux of the war. When you end the famines, your body can comfortably make adjustments to let go of the insurance fat it stored to prepare for upcoming famines. Once the famines are gone for good, your body can readapt by getting rid of fat that has become mal-adaptive. Your body and you have a new need, to use up the fat it doesn't need anymore.

The way to do this is coming up, but first let's take a look at some other factors that really influence your weight, and then some long-held beliefs that may be holding you back but are just plain untrue.

# CHAPTER 3

## What We Don't Know for Sure

### Famine Sensitivity

Is obesity inherited? You may believe it is, based on the prevalence of overweight people in your family, or a neighbor's family. A relationship appears rather obvious because overweight parents have kids who are or become overweight more often than not. And research bears this out.

When an overweight person says she's "got her mother's body," she is telling the truth from a certain perspective. But when she says this, she probably doesn't really understand why this is true—what role heredity actually plays. People do not inherit obesity per se. But they do inherit a predisposing factor that makes it *more likely* that they will grow heavier by the year. *Famine sensitivity* plays a definite role in the feast or famine cycle. As we saw in Chapter 2, this factor influences the degree to which a body responds to a famine.

Obesity researchers Stephen O'Rahilly and I. Sadaf Farooqi said, "Hereditary influences on adiposity are profound and continuing."

In another study, T.T. Foch and C.W. Mclaren stated, "Obesity appears to be highly heritable, as determined by studies of twins and adoptees. If neither parent is obese, the likelihood of the child's becoming obese is only 8%. If one parent is obese, the likelihood jumps to 40%, and if both parents are overweight, the probability of the child's becoming obese is an astonishing 80%." These are statistics from obesity research, and they are frightening. Are kids from overweight parents just doomed to become fat and stay that way, no matter what they do?

## A Predisposition is Not a Cause

As we discussed in the last chapter, all human beings come into the world with various adaptive potentials—unique abilities to adjust to environmental stresses. We have been talking about the stress of inadequate food and this stress affects different people to different degrees. The degree to which a body reacts to the lack of food—famine sensitivity—is inherited. For some bodies, a restricted food intake doesn't affect them much, and they tolerate it well without serious changes in hunger, eating or metabolic rate. But, some bodies are at the other end of the scale. They react strongly to food deprivation with slowed metabolism and increased appetite with cravings. Bodies that react least have low famine sensitivity and bodies that react strongly to going hungry have high famine sensitivity. Most bodies are probably somewhere on a scale between these extremes, but it is likely that most human beings fall above the midpoint—with higher than average famine sensitivity. This is because of the important role that famine sensitivity has played in keeping humans alive for eons.

## The Whole Equation

Famine sensitivity by itself does not make anybody fat. But, famine sensitivity plus regular famines does. People with low famine sensitivity seem to be able to eat whatever they want, whenever they want. They normally don't binge or overeat as a result of missing a meal. They just fit eating into their lives when it's convenient. The erratic food supply of our modern environment doesn't cause them to gain weight, at least while they are young, because their bodies tolerate these famines so well. They just stay thin. But in a real serious famine, they may be at a higher risk for starvation.

Those with high famine sensitivity—a predisposition to gaining weight easily when intermittent under eating occurs—usually start gaining as a result of some type of restricted eating in their lives. This typically happens in grade school or high school. School schedules interfere with kids' ability to eat when they get hungry, and they have the type of bodies that adapt quickly to this stress. When they finally eat after going hungry for too long, they tend to overeat to make up for the famine. Their metabolisms get sluggish, they crave junk foods and they may start to binge.

You can determine your famine sensitivity just by looking at your own weight and diet history and then your close relatives: parents, siblings, aunts and uncles.

There is one more trait that makes a person more vulnerable to obesity. It is a special ability to tolerate going hungry. For some people, going hungry is not particularly uncomfortable. They don't have strong urges to seek food when they get hungry and can put off eating for long periods of time. Famines are easy for them. Unlike famine sensitivity, this trait is probably acquired as a result of erratic eating habits.

## High Famine Sensitivity of Racial Groups

According to the Center for Disease Control, several racial groups in the United States have especially high rates of obesity. This is a function of high famine sensitivity. They are African Americans, Hispanics and American Indians. The high rates of obesity and diabetes in these groups reflect the overall high famine sensitivity. Within a culture of habitual recurrent under eating, plus excessive make-up food, these subgroups are even more vulnerable than the general population.

Most people become more famine sensitive with age. This contributes to the gradual weight gain of most adults. Usually, they attribute this added weight to a decrease in metabolic rate and activity level, which may also add to weight gain, but increased famine sensitivity and poor regular eating habits also play a significant role.

## Tasha

Tasha is a 26-year-old African American woman who was 65 pounds overweight by her thirtieth birthday. She was tall and athletic and carried herself well, but the extra pounds bothered her, especially because her mother had diabetes and had been obese all her life. Tasha wanted to change that for herself.

Tasha started gaining weight in third grade. She became self-conscious and started to worry about getting fat like her mother. By fifth grade, she was teased and stopped eating lunch at school. She didn't tell her mother but when she got home she was ravenous and ate plenty. In spite of her many attempts to control her weight-gain, Tasha continued to gain throughout high school and into her 20s. She had no idea her ethnicity-related high famine sensitivity and her dieting were behind her struggle.

So, your famine sensitivity sets you up to gain weight, more or less, as a result of dieting. If you have high famine sensitivity and you have dieted off and on for many years, your weight problem is bound to be significant. But, you might be only moderately overweight, if your famine sensitivity is low, even if you have been a long-term dieter.

## Food Addiction

An 18-year veteran of at least ten diet programs, Joy actually referred to herself as a "professional dieter." Having lost several hundred pounds over the years, Joy had the weight loss part down pat. Her trouble, like everybody else, was staying there. Following one successful diet, Joy's group celebrated her success for reaching her weight loss goal of 65 pounds in just nine months. Joy received congratulations all around and felt a flush of pride at her accomplishment. Of course, she would keep the weight off this time—she had worked so hard, right down to the last two days before the weigh-in when she ate nothing but crackers and tea in order to make her goal. As Joy left the meeting, a thought struck her, *Why not stop at the bakery? I've been so good. A donut won't hurt. I deserve a little reward.* The next thing she knew, Joy was sitting in her car in her driveway, shoving donuts into her mouth, swallowing them so fast she thought she might choke. Finishing the 12-pack, Joy knew she was addicted to food. She couldn't find any other explanation for her behavior.

Some people sure act like food addicts. Maybe you're one of those who've earned the diagnosis. But, recall the research with starved normal weight volunteers that showed that these thin individuals experienced total preoccupation with food as well as other symptoms typically experienced by dieters, like cravings for fat producing foods, general apathy and depression. It appears that starvation provokes serious physical and psychological symptoms and that you can actually produce the symptoms of "food addiction" in people who are not and

43

never have been addicted to food, by starving them for a while. If one definition of addiction focuses on the development of withdrawal symptoms, then really, wouldn't we all be considered food addicts? Certainly, everyone would suffer withdrawal if food were withheld. And wouldn't just about anyone who was half-starved, when food was finally there, be liable to overeat, even binge?

How did the idea of food addiction get started? It is a relatively new notion. The term didn't exist until dieting took a firm hold on our culture. Today, food addiction is a favorite term overweight people and even professionals use to diagnose people who eat too much, binge, and choose all the "wrong" food. Many of us have been taught that obese people eat too much because they are addicted to food, unlike people who don't eat too much. Although it's a handy diagnosis to use to explain seemingly inexplicable behavior, food addiction is a misleading idea. The term is especially useful for thin people who have never experienced the typical diet cycle and all the crazy, compulsive eating that go with it.

## Emotional Overeating

Sally had dieted off and on for nearly 14 years. She was positive she was addicted to chocolate, and to sweets in general. Whenever she went through a disappointment, emotional struggle or frustration, she found herself eating boxes of chocolate chip cookies, pints of ice cream, candy bars and M&Ms. With the help of multitudes of diet gurus and movie star bingers, she concluded that she was a classic emotional overeater.

Multitudes embrace this false explanation for overeating, including famous people. The theory behind emotional overeating seems logical because bouts of bingeing are often accompanied by emotional distress of some kind. But do heavy emotions and excessive eating really have a direct cause/effect relationship? Just because they show up at about the same time doesn't necessarily mean one causes the other. Well, what about the multitudes of testimonies about emotional upheaval and terrific binges? Just one visit to any diet support group will convince you that there is indeed a relationship between these experiences. Most dieters will attest to a tendency to overeat under stress or heavy emotions. The evidence is so overwhelming, how can anyone deny it?

## Events That Trigger Overeating

We've established that dieters can only restrict their food intake for so long before they lose control of their eating. Overeating during the rebound phase is often accompanied by heavy emotions— discouragement, anger, fear, hopelessness, etc. It appears that emotional triggers play a part in diet rebound, and often, dieters fall off their diet wagon abruptly around some significant emotional event. But whether a loss of control happens gradually or suddenly, emotions are usually blamed. There is a reason for the connection but it's not what you think.

What are these "significant emotional events" that often occur coincidentally with dieters' overeating?

- Loss of a loved one or change in a relationship (positive or negative)
- Injury or illness—the person or others
- Cruise or vacation
- Promotion or demotion
- Move or construction
- Financial distress/improvement
- Marriage and/or marriage struggles or divorce
- Threat—physical or psychological
- New relationship/relationship problem, crisis

- Serious disappointment or argument/making up
- Rejection, perceived rejection
- Remark about person or weight
- Having a baby

Notice that this list reflects the major stresses for people in general, some positive and some negative. We all go through these things as part of life. New research has recently been done showing a positive link between *happiness* and overeating. It looks like we can't feel anything without finding ourselves in front of the refrigerator. But what really causes some people to overeat when they experience these stresses and the feelings they inspire?

## Two Groups of People Experience All Kinds of Stress and Emotional Trouble in Two Distinct Ways:

### 1. "Well-Fed People"

I'll call the first type "well-fed people." These are people who eat enough food pretty much whenever they need to eat. They are not dieters. They do not avoid food because they are not afraid of food and they are not worried about getting fat. In fact, they like food. So, they eat and never have much trouble with it.

When "well-fed people" face any kind of significant stress (even a positive one), they tend to experience a loss of appetite, at least temporarily. This is natural. When their boss calls them in to the office and they know what's going to happen, they might even feel nauseated, but they definitely aren't looking forward to lunch! And when a boyfriend, a great boyfriend, says to the "well-fed girl" that he needs "space," it's not likely that she'll go right home and eat a quart of rocky road ice cream. This is not because she isn't having heavy emotions. It's because she couldn't eat if you paid her. She's upset, not hungry. These examples illustrate the normal response to stress: temporary depressed appetite and food avoidance.

Think about it. If your body has to deal with external pressures, changes and challenges that force adaptations, it goes on heightened alert. Eating is, in a way, stressful to bodies because it requires energy and causes the alert, focused aspects of your physical self to slow down. So eating, and especially eating a lot when stressed, is counterproductive. Naturally, "well-fed people" don't do it.

## 2. Dieters

Unlike "well-fed people" who eat on demand, dieters are often under fed: hungry, or over-hungry. Their chronic under-satisfied hunger causes dieters who experience heavy emotions and/or stress to actually have two serious problems: one is the emotional stress and the other is their under-satisfied hunger. This combination sets dieters' bodies up for an interesting challenge to adapt to both stresses.

Instead of appetite suppression under the influence of an external stress, underfed bodies experience a paradoxical response. The underfed dieter experiences a surge in appetite and often a loss of control over eating as a result of the stress encounter. This makes it appear that the stress caused the overeating, but since "well-fed people" do not overeat under the influence of stress, something else must be involved. That something else is under-satisfied hunger—a stress in itself, which bodies are capable of solving through biochemical influence. That leaves only the remaining emotional stress to cope with.

## Non-Dieters, Too

Remember that non-dieters also experience famines when they eat recklessly and become over-hungry. They are vulnerable to overeating from emotional cues, often just as susceptible as dieters.

In conclusion, so-called emotional overeating is not about the emotions or the stress; it's about dieting, going hungry and adaptation.

So, there are very real reasons that people overeat under the influence of emotional stress, but it isn't what we've always thought. If it were true that emotions directly cause overeating and bingeing, everyone would do it. There'd be no hope for any of us. Let's face it, we're emotional creatures and life will always be fraught with heavy emotions and stress. If there really is a cause/effect relationship between these two experiences, we are all predestined to overeating and consequent weight problems just for being human.

Understanding the true relationship among these experiences— undereating, emotional stress, and overeating—leads to hope and confidence. First of all, dieters can get out from under the fear that stress and emotional struggles doom them to binges and weight gain. And as they change their eating patterns, their response to stress will normalize—they will experience a loss of appetite rather than a surge. This shift is hard for dieters to imagine, dieters who have reacted to emotional upheavals with binges for years. But when it happens, what a relief!

## Carbohydrate Addiction

Now here's a theory that really packs some logic! What do people binge on? Steak? Chicken? Fish? Vegetables? Fruits? Hardly. Although vegetables are mostly carbs, dieters usually do not crave or binge on them. It isn't really practical because, pound for pound, vegetables don't fill you up before you get sick of them. Fruits are mostly carbs too, but again, I have never known a dieter to crave apples much. Meats and fish do have calories and fat, but again, dieters don't tend to binge on these high-protein foods. They seem to have built-in satiety limits, unlike simple carbohydrate foods.

Back to the question: What do people binge on? Of course, mostly carbohydrate foods, the ones that are baked, processed, refined, sweetened, laced with chocolate, and go so well with ice cream. In fact, the latest poll on the eating habits of Americans found that bakery products head the list of foods that we ingest the most. Really? Scary.

So, it does seem logical that many people are "carbohydrate addicted." And, dieters appear to be particularly so. Processed and refined carbohydrate foods are usually the focus of dieters' binges. They crave and tend to binge on cakes, candy, muffins, pastries, chocolates, cookies, ice cream, chips, and French fries, to name a few favorites. But is this really an addiction, or is there another variable in the equation?

The question to ask is: Why do dieters particularly favor these refined, calorie-rich foods? It's not because they don't care and it's not because they don't know any better. They eat these high sugar and carb-loaded foods because they crave them because they *need* them. They need fat and the best ingredient necessary for making fat is sugar, some form of carbohydrate. It is their bodies' efficient system for recovering from the diet famines they impose and restocking the fat for the next famine. Other types of foods like proteins and vegetables and fruits just don't do the trick nearly as well.

## Not So Fast

Very rapid weight loss is still the mainstream approach to weight loss in our country. People continue to believe they can lose 80 pounds in six months that took 25 them years to gain. But if you talk to a trainer, a dietician or a nutritionist, you'll usually find at least some resistance to quick weight-loss plans, even ones backed by medical professionals. These experts have long been involved with dieters and quick weight-loss gimmicks. They have learned by personal experience that people need to eat *enough good food to lose weight slowly.*

Although tiny cracks in the eat-less-exercise-more paradigm are surfacing among some health professionals, plenty of diet propaganda continues to show up everywhere—television, the Internet, billboards, even in your mailbox. Just think about the rag magazines at the grocery store check out. "Lose 20 pounds the first two weeks!" "How I lost 85 pounds in five months!" "Lose up to 50 pounds in six weeks!" Have you believed these claims in the past? Have you managed to lose a lot of weight in a short period of time just as these people describe—more than once? Were you happier as a thinner person? And were you devastated when the weight came back?

I know what you're thinking. You're thinking, *I've known for a long time that these diets don't work for me, or if they ever did, the weight loss didn't last that long. So, now I'm finding out why the diets backfire and how my survival mechanisms have caused me to gain weight. Great—I believe you. So now what do I do?*

Hold on, we're getting there.

# PART II

## Discovering Your
## Body for a Change

# CHAPTER 4

## Fixing Broken Body Signals

Body signals are built-in communication systems between you and your body that help you know what's going on—what your body needs. Our bodies send us these signals to get essential needs met for optimal performance.

Here are a few examples of body signals: thirst, hunger, fullness, urge to eliminate waste, dangers like burning heat or cold, lack of oxygen, and all pain signals. The central nervous system manages all these body signals, coordinates priorities and keeps informed of what's going on. Without body signals, we wouldn't know how to take care of our bodies which would definitely lead to trouble. When we ignore our body signals, that leads to trouble, too.

As dieters, we learn to ignore hunger. If we *learn* to ignore hunger at some point, we must have been paying attention to our hunger naturally at some earlier time.

## Body Signals When We Were Kids

Babies and children are naturally in tune with their hunger and let their caregivers know they need food without fail. They are not inhibited by anything—time, place, inconvenience, the last meal, or whether anybody else is hungry. Kids just automatically seek food whenever they get the urge to eat. It's how their bodies are designed. Kids don't know about calories or fat grams or sugar or carbohydrates or what protein is all about. They know when they're hungry and they know what they like, and they know when they're full, period. These simple truths account for the freedom they experience to eat and enjoy food. If they are consistently fed decent food on time, they will continue to enjoy this natural, in-born freedom.

## How do kids get away from this natural way of eating?

There was a time when you ate like a baby, like a kid. You lived in perfect harmony with your body's hunger signals. What happened? Something began to interfere with your ability to eat on time. Maybe it was school or day care. Maybe after-school activities like athletics or dance. These schedule conflicts with your body's need for fuel often interfered with your eating on time. You may have noticed this, struggling with your unmet hunger needs, but maybe not. Sometimes, bodies are so adaptive that hunger simply takes a backseat to "more important" issues, like soccer. And, parents usually don't realize how important eating on time really is. They may think, *Going hungry can't hurt anybody.* But it can, and it does.

## Sherrie

Sherrie was a little chubby by the time she was 6. She'd been plump ever since she started preschool. Concerned about her daughter's weight,

Sherrie's mother signed her up for dancing lessons on Saturdays and soccer every day after school. With a weight problem herself, Sherrie's mom did not want her daughter to suffer with it, too. She kept Sherrie's breakfast fat free with cereal and skim milk, and just brought water for the soccer practice. Sherrie complained that she was hungry midway through her dancing lesson, but her mother thought that was a good sign and promised a lunch when the lesson finished. Usually hungry after school, Sherrie again protested that she was hungry at soccer practice, but she was only able to drink juice until the end of the physically intense hour. Sherrie grew more muscular—and fatter, too.

When and however you began to lose touch with your hunger, if you are famine sensitive, you probably began to gain weight. Look back now to the time that you first noticed you were overweight. If you were not dieting, which automatically interferes with natural eating, what was your life like then? For most, eating was being squeezed out some of the time. Children would never willingly do this. So, there are two major ways to get out of touch with your body's fuel needs; accidentally, when schedules interfere with eating on time, and deliberately, when well-meaning mothers, or fathers or caregivers, interfere with eating on purpose.

The times people are particularly vulnerable to losing touch with their hunger and fullness signals are; school, sports and after-school activities, peer pressure during adolescence, introduction to dieting at any time, job pressures and poor food availability, having a baby, and major stresses that interfere with normal appetite.

## Looking for Hunger in All the Possible Places

So what does "real" hunger feel like? This may be the question of the century for you. Most dieters say they are either never hungry or always hungry. They have the urge to eat but are not really hungry. These are symptoms of the feast or famine cycle. *Getting back in touch with your genuine hunger is the first key to permanent weight loss.* Especially at the beginning, it is absolutely necessary that your hunger signals guide your eating. This connection will enable you to get off the feast or famine cycle.

Always eating in response to your definite hunger signals is the habit that sends the message to your body that famines are things of the past; there is now no need to continue adapting to famines by storing fat. Eating on time interrupts the feast or famine cycle; ending famines, ending overeating, ending bingeing and cravings for fat-producing foods. And you'll be able to finally enjoy exercise. These changes end adaptive weight gain.

## What Hunger Feels Like

Remember when you were a child playing outside in the summer, and you suddenly became hungry. Maybe you were very hungry. What was that feeling? You just knew it. "Hey Mom, I'm hungry!" It was an empty feeling. It was an urge. It interrupted your play because it felt so strong. You noticed and identified it easily because it was compelling—a good feeling in a way because you knew there was food.

Hunger can be that way again; simple, strong, easy to identify, a good feeling to be satisfied well. You don't have to debate about it. You don't have to analyze it. You don't have to ignore it! You don't have to fear it. In fact, your hunger is the key to getting a normal relationship with food again, just like when you were a kid.

## The Very Best Appetite Suppressant

In our mad quest to get around our hunger, we've developed and manufactured and discovered hundreds of appetite suppressants. These various products and methods of curtailing or eliminating our appetites is wildly popular because of the rampant belief that hunger is the enemy of weight loss. But just like the tens of thousands of other popular diet products, these methods of squelching hunger are doomed to fail as lasting weight loss aids. Somehow bodies manage to eventually work around them and get their survival needs met. Actually, the very best appetite suppressant, and the only one you can safely take indefinitely, is food. This is a big relief to dieters who learn to get in touch with their hunger again. They have tried just about everything, including disgusting-tasting power bars and shakes, to get rid of their hunger without eating real food. Usually the idea of suppressing their appetite by actually eating food seems preposterous at first. *Are you kidding, using food to suppress my appetite?* Yes! We've been blind to this fact because we've always thought that food is *the enemy* of overweight people. But now we know that's not true.

## So, How Exactly Do You Get in Touch With Your Hunger?

Once you decide that hunger is your friend and that you need to re-establish your relationship with your body's hunger signals, invite your body to let you know when it needs fuel. And listen for these signals, reminding yourself that they are the key to normalizing your relationship with food and eventually getting a normal body. Much of the recovery of body communication depends on your understanding of why you're doing it. If you are confident that tuning in to your body signals and *working with them* holds the key to your freedom to eat like a normal person and gradually lose weight that will stay off, then you are probably going to do well. But if you are unsure that you can trust your body and stay out of touch, then you may find this step difficult.

Sometimes, hunger feels like weakness, or breathlessness. Others describe hunger feelings as "the bottom falling out." Stomach gurgling is a signal for some but meaningless for others. Headache, and irritability, may signal hunger, especially when coupled with caffeine. Thoughts of foods, or sweets, can mean it's time to eat. An "empty" feeling is the signal for some. Thoughts of specific foods can signal hunger. This isn't a definitive list. You may have other cues that your body needs fuel.

### How do you know you are really hungry and not just wanting to eat for pleasure?

As you know, cravings for pleasure foods—poor quality fat producers— are often a signal that your body needs to do some make-up eating. Strong interest in these foods reflects a famine in the past, usually the recent past. So while you're dreaming about chocolate chip cookies, *take a look at your recent eating behavior*—the past day or two. Pleasure-oriented eating is a symptom, not a judgment of your character. So if you've gotten overly hungry recently, just learn from it. On the other hand, if you're thinking about cookies or chocolate it may be because you are just plain hungry—really hungry for good food.

Once you get off the feast or famine cycle, the type of food you want can give you information about your overall eating patterns. If you want some eggs and toast and OJ, or a Caesar salad with shrimp, or a bowl of oatmeal with nuts, you can be pretty sure you just need to eat. If you've just eaten a wonderful side of delicious pasta with a salad, and you want a piece of cheesecake, two things may be going on. The first one is the possibility of make-up eating. You may feel full, but there's always room for more when you have been under eating recently. The second possibility is that you just want the cheesecake because you love the taste of cheesecake. Once you are off the feast or famine cycle you might still want cheesecake, but you won't *need* it. It will be easy to pass up or just have a bite of a shared piece. No kidding.

## Rating Your Hunger

This is an invaluable skill you will use throughout your recovery from the diet cycle. When you are just starting out, rating your hunger will help you learn about your hunger. Use a scale from 1 to 10—1 being just a quiet hint of hunger and 10 when you are blind with starvation. Naturally, you are going to avoid the high numbers. But when is the best hunger level to start eating? At 3? At 5? The immediacy of your response to your hunger will be strict at the beginning of your recovery, say a 2 or 3, but it will relax a bit as you and your body gets into a rhythm together. You may be so used to getting very hungry before you eat, at an 8 or 9 that this might be a bit of a shock.

## What does hunger say?

Your body's hunger tells you it is low on fuel and possibly what *kind* of fuel it needs at the moment. Interpreting these signals accurately takes some practice. Bodies need calories and specific nutrients. You can tell when your body needs particular nutrients by your interest in certain foods. Just as you craved sugar and fat as a dieter, eating good food on time will be accompanied by new cravings—for baked beans, or bananas, or salads or oranges or avocados—real food. The idea that our bodies can actually communicate their nutritional needs this way may seem pretty far-fetched, until you turn the reins over to your body and eat the great quality food that really looks good to you for a change. It's amazing.

## The Other Important Body Signal

Isn't it interesting that this signal—fullness—isn't the first one we've talked about? There's a reason for that. The fullness or satisfaction signal is quite dependent on how well the hunger signal is satisfied—how good the food is and how well you have been eating recently. You can't succeed without skills in both categories. When you are on the feast or famine cycle and you ignore your hunger or can't satisfy it because of other limitations, you are going to have trouble with your fullness signals too. And if you don't learn to read your body's fuel-full signal, you'll block your body's new need to adapt through weight loss.

Ex-dieters struggle with this signal. This is because of their history of going hungry and then overeating. Dieting really messes with your satisfied signals because without adequate food, your body is forced to override the fullness sensations to get any extra fuel it can to make up for the calorie deficit. When your body adjusts your sense of fullness, expanding it really, your body makes it possible to take in extra fuel to store up for the future. So, after you've had a "good week" of dieting, and you feel full following a meal, those three bites of chicken cacciatore still look good. A dozen rationalizations go through your head as you finish the dish. You feel stuffed, but don't blame the great cooking.

Like tuning in to your hunger, getting the "'stop" cue will take some time and practice. Sometimes at the beginning, you'll go over and eat a bit too much. In time this will feel uncomfortable, which is the normal response to becoming over-full. When you were dieting, at times you felt compelled to go on eating after you felt full, but when you are eating enough every time you get hungry, you will want to avoid this over-full feeling. If you continue to get over full regularly as you get off the cycle, it's important to decide to push your plate away a bit *before* you feel satisfied. This will not be difficult for you. You and your body may need a little extra support in learning what satisfied feels like.

## The One Bite Threshold

Have you ever seen a baby in a high chair eating off a spoon? At first, the baby's wide- open mouth eagerly slurps up the applesauce from the spoon his mother offers. One spoon, two, three, he opens his mouth wide and she glides it in. Then, about the eighth spoonful, he turns his head away as the spoon comes towards him. His mother scoops the leftover applesauce off his face and tries again. But the baby closes his mouth and throws his arm up at the spoon coming after him. If Mother manages to sneak another bite into the baby's mouth, he spits it out. The mother may try again and again, but the baby is done with applesauce.

What's this got to do with fullness for overweight people? The same instinctive fuel-full signals that babies have, you can have too. This is your goal; to get so tuned in to your body's satisfaction signals that you can sense, within one bite, when to stop eating. When that happens, it gets a lot easier to trust your body. I have had the experience of having to spit out a last bite when I miscalculated. That's how sensitive you can become.

## FAQs

### I never want to stop eating, so how can I trust my body to tell me I'm full?

According to Webster, *full* means having eaten all the food that one wants. Doesn't that sound crazy, dangerous, impossible? Really? *All the food one wants?* But this is the definition and the experience we're after. While you are still on the feast or famine cycle, your fullness signals are probably going to be all messed up. This is because adaptation doesn't suddenly shift when you start to change your eating. Your intermittent dieting has warped your fullness signals, so you may seldom or never feel the urge to stop eating *at first*. But remember, the clear full signal depends on your eating enough good food on time. First, you must learn to identify your hunger, and as you do that better—consistently satisfying your hunger, your fullness signals will become better defined. Then, you'll be able to know, without a doubt, that you are satisfied and you will want to stop eating more food, and you will be able to cut your intake gradually because your body will be ready. Honestly, this is how it works

## Do you have to eat slowly to know you're full?

This idea is based on the concept that your fullness signals may be delayed, so you have to wait for them to catch up with your eating, otherwise you'll overeat before you know it. This principle is probably linked to the symptoms of the feast or famine cycle. As a dieter, your body signals are affected by the under eating that goes with the conscious eating-avoidance pattern. And your fuel-full signals become vague—you don't know whether you are full or not, so you don't know whether or not you should keep eating.

The solution to this dilemma, diet programs suggest, is to eat very slowly or stop eating and wait for your fullness signals to show up. Perhaps this is a good technique for dieters, but it is not usually necessary when you get off the diet cycle and tune in consistently to your hunger and fullness. The majority of people who stop dieting and get off the feast or famine cycle have no need to eat at an artificially slow pace, unless they want to. Many report wolfing down a sandwich because they have little time, but stopping with three bites left because they suddenly *know* they are full. Sometimes, it is just necessary to eat more quickly, but when your body is in control, you will know when you are full. Just pay attention! At the right time, you will not want any more to eat, so naturally you will stop eating. Your body knows how to do this. If over time you discover that your satisfaction signal is delayed, then you know what to do.

## Questions of the Millennia

Don't you have to eat less than you're using up to lose weight?

Yes, you do.

You know the equation: X in - Y out = net gain or loss. If X is the energy input (food) and Y is the energy output (metabolism + activity), and X is greater than Y, then weight gain would result, all other factors being the same. And if Y is greater than X, a net weight loss would result. It's a simplified equation but it's useful to see a picture of this principle. It's the basic formula for every kind of weight loss—this one too.

But traditional diets are designed just one way: they *force* bodies to give up muscle and fat reserves by imposing a sudden and serious calorie deficit. *Forcing* bodies to get along on less food so abruptly and so drastically is the crux of the problem. It is where the war begins—an unwinnable war.

Well, if you're satisfying your hunger every time you get hungry, how can you possibly lose weight? Won't your eating keep up with your metabolism and activity level?

If forcing your body to get along on less food is the problem in traditional diets, how do you eat less food by eating whenever you're hungry? Your body isn't going to do this voluntarily, right? Not exactly, but you're getting warm. The question boils down to this: how to eat less than your body is using without tripping your body's survival response?

You do it very carefully.

## Helping Your Body *Need* to Lose Weight

The other way to eat less food than you're burning up doesn't involve forcing your body to suddenly struggle on less food, violating its survival needs. It's what we've been talking about all along—it's about changing your body's food supply so it can change its need for fat. When you do that over time, getting securely off the feast or famine fat-producing cycle, your body will *allow you to gradually take in less food so it can use up your extra fat.* It will do this by making biochemical adjustments as you change your eating patterns and food choices.

What? You mean to tell me that my body will *need to lose weight?*

That's exactly what I said. When you get off the cycle that has kept your fat going, you can then back off on your food intake. Your body will cooperate with your effort to lose weight because it is not in a protracted famine environment any more. You'll know you are avoiding the war with your body as long as you stay free from the symptoms of the cycle. You will, by cooperating with your body, actually invite your body to stop storing fat and then gradually start burning it up by making non-threatening adjustments in your eating. You and your body will finally have a chance to lose weight together—for good! The specifics on this recovery plan are coming up.

It is very important to know that your body will need your help and cooperation in making decisions about what, when and how much to eat. Recovery doesn't happen by accident simply because people start to eat better food. It's a bit more complicated than that, but armed with determination and a good mind, you can do it as many have.

**Benefits**

Although weight loss by these principles isn't immediate, there are many early advantages to eating according to your body signals and getting off the yo-yo diet cycle. Some report these experiences within a week or two. Others a little while longer, but all report these advantages.

1. Calming and normalization of appetite
2. Clearer definition of hunger and fullness
3. Increased desire for better-quality foods
4. Improved sense of well-being, self-esteem
5. Increased energy
6. Decrease in guilt, shame about eating and hunger
7. Intolerance for going hungry
8. Improved mood

The long-term perks are just as wonderful and are coming up in Part III.

***What* You Know About Food**

As a dieter, you probably learned a lot about food. Some of the information you've learned may be helpful in your recovery from dieting. But some of the prejudices you've learned will only work against you. There's one thing you have learned about food from this book: not enough of it causes some serious problems for you and your body.

Let's go back to the basics. Overeating, by itself, is not the problem. Food alone is not the problem. The problem is dieting, overeating, lousy food and the *pattern of eating*—the feast or famine cycle—that cause people to gain and maintain extra weight.

We've talked about when to eat. We've talked about how much to eat to get off the cycle. Now we have to discuss what to eat and this is just as important as the other two. *What* do you eat in order to recover and lose weight for good? To put it most succinctly, you eat really good food. That's it. I know I'd better define my terms here—you may be unsure about exactly what that means. Let's talk about food!

# CHAPTER 5

## Let's Eat!

### What You Eat

So far, we've spent a lot of time on body signals—hunger and fullness—and these message systems are vital to your recovery. Your body holds the key to your weight loss by virtue of these communication systems, and you will need to cooperate with them in order to succeed. So what kinds of foods will be best in this cooperative effort?

Actually, *what you eat* is your diet and your diet is what you eat. The word "diet" has become synonymous with food restriction, exercise and weight loss, but the simplest definition of diet is *what you eat*, whether making any effort to lose weight or not. Diets usually spell out a number of restrictions of what and especially how much you are allowed to eat in order to lose weight. Often, restrictions involve carbohydrates, or sugar or flour or white flour or fats or sweets or red meat or whatever. Eliminating certain foods and food groups is often artificial and unrealistic for the long run. Although basic dietary principles may be at work in some programs, there is almost no end to the creativity of diet organizations and authors in restricting dieters' appetites in new ways. Because of the universal effect of limiting caloric intake, most of the popular approaches do result in weight loss, at least for a while.

It's amazing the number of prejudices people have about food. There have been so many theories and discoveries and diet programs over the pat 60 years. Consequently, almost everybody in our culture suffers from unfounded notions about food. As a dieter, you have probably learned a lot about food, but maybe you've missed some important information. You may have learned that certain foods or food groups are "good" and others are "bad," but these prejudices are usually untrue, and since traditional diets are based on the sudden and unrealistic restriction of calories, foods that are perfectly fine in a balanced diet may be restricted or not even allowed. Some of the diet guidelines might help in encouraging higher quality eating, and that is really important, but the serious restriction of overall food intake makes it impossible to stay on track indefinitely.

## The Latest in a Long Line

Beverly learned about the HCG diet from a friend who'd been on it and lost 22 pounds in a month. She got very excited about it because she'd been dieting for 10 years and thought she'd finally found the solution to her struggle. She bought the required hormones and began the 500-calorie-a-day regimen. (I've always wondered why you need the hormones.) The diet allowed Beverly a small serving of a protein food, a vegetable, a bread and a fruit. She stayed on the restrictive diet for almost two months! This took almost superhuman strength, she said as she looked back on it. Beverly lost 18 pounds and felt terrible, although she certainly looked thinner.

Then, Beverly simply lost the will to go on starving herself. She couldn't take it anymore; it wasn't worth it, she said. So, she began to eat, and eat, and eat. She said she ate everything, almost, she said, including inanimate objects! She gained the weight back as fast as she had lost it, but the ride down on the scale and then back up was grueling. She said she wished she had never heard of the HCG diet.

There are two things going on here. Beverly's calorie intake is severely restricted, but there's another kind of deficit for which diets are notorious; most are rigid in disallowing dieters to be sensitive to their bodies' appetite fluctuations from day to day, for both type and amount of food. Bodies on a diet are usually in a food straight jacket. Dieters committed to specific diet plans are rarely allowed to have any flexibility regarding what and how much they eat: Bodies not only don't get as much food as they need, they are also very restricted to specific foods without regard for their food interests and needs. So, before we talk about exactly what foods are recommended here, there's another important thing to learn in order to understand the program you can live with.

**Variety and Balance**

There are natural fluctuations in our appetites and our interest in various foods. You doubt this? Try eating eggs three meals a day, every day, and watch what happens to your appetite for eggs. Variety in your diet is important for ensuring that you'll eat a broad range of nutrients over time. As we know, foods are made up of different nutrients and calorie sources like proteins, carbohydrates and fats. And we've noted that there is a connection between the types of food you're interested in eating and the food your body needs. If certain foods are limited or restricted in a diet, bodies may miss these nutrient sources and the dieter might develop a strong interest in these foods. On the other hand, when diets promote some food types as preferable over others, dieters may end up with an aversion to such foods. So, we need variety in our diets, to be sure. This is why restaurants have menus, I suppose. Naturally, the same types of food over and over just don't appeal to us.

The point is, your appetite for certain foods is a general a reflection of what you've been eating, or not eating, and if it's off-kilter, you can fix it. If you've eliminated certain high quality foods or food groups, reintroducing them will bring you back into balance. And if you've focused your diet on a particular quality food group, like protein, back off and get that food group back to a balanced place in your diet.

## Bad Food, Worse Food, and Totally Evil Food

My work with ex-dieters in recovery has often felt like deprogramming members of a cult. They seem to have been brainwashed about food, as well as eating, portions, hunger, appetite, cravings, calories, carbs, fat and why they overeat. It is challenging to uproot long-held beliefs and prejudices, especially when they are associated with anxiety about food in general. Why do we have so much confusion about weight and eating in our culture? Most of it comes from diet propaganda and even medical research. We have new studies, new information, new cautions, new guidelines, new techniques and new diets every week. And after a time, there are new reports refuting all that went before.

This deprogramming process is often my main role in coaching, but my power to break through years of prejudice is limited. People must be willing to let go of these long- held beliefs and embrace a whole new way of thinking about food and eating. If they can't do this, they will be unable to break free of the war with their bodies. Ultimately, I am not the deprogrammer, they are.

## Calories

Calories are good. Let's say that one more time: ***Calories are good!*** We couldn't get along without them for very long. We need calories. Calories are units of energy that may or may not come along with various nutrients. We especially need nutrient-loaded calories. We call the calories in products like pop "empty calories" because they don't have any nutrients besides sugar. Fruits, on the other hand, although also made up of mostly water, contain important nutrients. So, there's a big difference between foods that are mostly water but supply only empty calories and water-based foods that are nutrient-loaded. It's essential that you focus your food choices on the nutrient-rich foods so all your valuable calories can count towards your recovery.

No-calorie, low-calorie, sugar-free, fat-free and low fat foods are not holy, and usually they are downright undesirable. Foods that fit these categories, so attractive to dieters, are chemically altered to taste like they are the real thing. But they aren't the real thing. They are artificially altered to mimic the real thing by adding chemicals, bulk agents, artificial sweetening agents, and fat substitutes while taking natural fat and sugar out. I call this artificial food, and it is all produced for a culture that is convinced that calories, fat, and sugar, by themselves, make people fat. They do not. Maladaptive eating patterns make people fat.

## Here We Go—FOOD!

The ultimate goal in developing your diet is to choose foods that are as close as possible to the way nature produced them. Simple foods prepared simply are best for quality and nutrition. Choose organic. It's always the best way to go if you have a choice and can afford it. If money is an issue, the most important foods to keep on your organic list are dairy, meat and eggs. If there is only one ingredient on certain foods, i.e. raspberries, you know they belong at the top of your grocery list.

There is a movement in this country toward fresh, whole, organic, vegetarian-based diets. This is an extremely important trend away from the processed, human-designed, additive-laden stuff that stocks much of our grocery store shelves. We all need to improve our diets, heading toward this type of food—clean food I call it—for our health and well being. Some people in recovery find going cold turkey to plant-based eating works best for them. *However,* I have discovered in my counseling that many people need to transition more gradually. Sometimes, inspired by one of these whole, vegetarian-type diets, ex-dieters try to change things all at once, and in doing that, set them selves up for failure. They try to go from hamburgers and French fries to kale and sunflower seeds in a day. Another problem is this abrupt change cuts their calorie intake so drastically that they just can't keep it up and the super quality eating shift goes to waste.

So, definitely decide now to move your diet towards plant-based eating, whenever you can. Perhaps you shouldn't change everything at once, but start by adding more fresh fruit and vegetables, whole grains, nuts, complex carbs, etc. to your diet. Carrying fresh foods with you for snacks and building meals around them at times will most likely ensure that you fit more of them into your eating, improving the quality of your diet every day.

There's one essential skill you'll need to keep your diet high in quality food: understanding food labels. This may have seemed complicated for you when you were looking for so many percentages and grams and calories in the past, but it's really not that hard to get the basics for good quality eating. When reading a label, the first thing to look for is simple: do you recognize the individual ingredients listed? If not, never mind. If the first ingredient starts with "organic" that's a good quality start, so read on. It's not a good sign to find many ingredients, perhaps over ten, unless they qualify as simple, recognizable foods. And it's certainly not a good sign if the label lists any word you can't pronounce. The best ingredient list is a short one that sounds familiar.

Because ingredients are listed in order of quantity, the first three or four really count. Avoid products with high fructose corn syrup (or anything that sounds like it), partially hydrogenated oils, trans-fats, sugar, and a lot of cholesterol. Beneficial fats include polyunsaturated fat, mono-saturated fat, and many plant-based oils. Some are better than others. Inclusion of protein, carbohydrate and fat is often an indication of a well-balanced food, such as cereal and yogurt.

**Broad Food Groups**

The first way to look at food is in three big categories. Sometimes foods bridge two categories but each of the divisions comes with a basic definition. The second way I've arranged food is by quality using a fuel analogy. People in recovery quickly get used to these categories. No one food, eaten on occasion, will determine whether or not an individual will recover her best weight and a normal relationship with food. But, foods considered poor quality, when eaten regularly, may keep a person stuck.

You may be surprised that the quality foods on the REAL FOOD list include just about every meal-type food you can think of. Formerly taboo foods like cheese, peanut butter and even butter make their way to the Real Food list. Of course, there are some practical things to consider about these fat-concentrated foods, and we'll cover these in just a minute.

## REAL FOOD

Real food is easy to define. It is good quality food or combinations thereof that are not overly laden with fat (particularly of the saturated or trans-types), or sugar or corn syrup. Now, there is nothing inherently wrong with fat or sugar. It's just that in quantity, they squeeze out quality nutrients and other important food ingredients like whole fruits and vegetables, lean protein and whole grain carbohydrates. The eater gets full on fatty and sugary foods without adequate nutrition—a quality famine. No, real food is generally simple—mixed greens salads accompanied by just about anything, grilled chicken (or non-meat protein), blueberries and goat cheese, stir-fry shrimp and vegetables with rice, eggs with toast and OJ, pork tenderloin, baked potatoes, broccoli, granola with almonds. It is not complicated to learn to eat real foods and leave the other stuff alone when you're eating enough.

In order to cover a broad spectrum of nutrients, food choices should enable variety and balance over time. Variety refers to eating food from all the food groups daily if possible, with emphasis on whole grains, fruits and vegetables, and lean-protein foods. This recommendation stems from the fact that most of us have poor habits where food variety, especially fresh, whole food, is concerned. You'll notice that the Real Food list is not focused on low fat. In my experience, popular low-fat diets usually leave a person unsatisfied and frequently hungry. This is because fat provides long-term blood sugar stability and an important feeling of fullness and satisfaction after eating. Besides, taking dietary fat to an artificially low level cuts calories dramatically, setting a dieter up for the feast or famine cycle and failure. Of course, a high-fat diet is no better, so good judgment is called for here.

## Dieting at the Grocery Store

It's possible, and even recommended, that the person determined to conquer her weight problem for good learn to *run* past certain aisles while shopping for real food at the grocery store. There is no need to linger in the chips or candy aisles, or the freezer laden with ice cream treats. The bakery section may beckon, but except for whole grain breads, it's off limits too. The reason is simple: *You won't eat food that isn't there.* And if you didn't buy it at the grocery store when you were in a strong, resolute mood, you will not have to cope with the temptation later at home.

## REAL FOOD LIST:

### *Fruits and Vegetables*
all fruits, fresh, frozen, canned in 100% juice
all vegetables, fresh, frozen, canned
vegetable-based dishes, such as oriental stir-fry, vegetable-based soups
fruit jams and jellies, all-fruit is better
juices, 100% unsweetened fruit or vegetable juice
salads, side dishes made from vegetables and/or fruits
soups made from real foods

### *Breads Nuts, Seeds, Legumes*
seeds of all types
nuts of all kinds
peanut butter, almond butter, other seed/nut spreads
beans, legumes of all kinds

### *Grains, Cereals*
*Whole-grain foods in this category are always best*
all unfrosted loaf-type breads, whole grain
bagels, English muffins, dinner rolls, pretzels, whole grain crackers

all unsweetened or very low sugar cold or hot cereals (sugar is OK as
a condiment)
pasta, all types, whole grain
rice, especially brown and wild
all sandwiches made with real food fillings (slip vegetables in here)
pizza with lighter cheese, no pizza meat, any vegetables
old world grains, i.e. quinoa, couscous

### *Dairy*
milk, whole or fat reduced
cheese, all types—this is essentially a condiment
cottage cheese
yogurt, the most natural kind you can find
cream as a condiment
sour cream, cream cheese
milk-based, soups
eggs

### *Meat, Poultry, Seafood*
beef, lean cuts
chicken, white meat preferred
fish, all types (wild caught is best)
turkey, other poultry, white meat preferred
ground beef, 95% lean
pork, lean cuts—tenderloin is great
shellfish
soups, stews
meat substitutes, i.e. tofu

### *Fats, spreads*
butter
vegetable oils, no trans fats, no margarine

## Condiments
mustard, vinegar, relishes
fresh or dried herbs, spices
sugar, syrup
ketchup, barbecue sauce, hot sauce, salsa
steak sauces
fruit dips, veggie dips
salad dressings
jelly, jams, preserves (real fruit is best)
mayonnaise, olive oil is best

## Beverages
unsweetened fruit or vegetable juice, all-juice pops
sugar-free beverages, diet pop, powdered drinks—additives, not recommended
milk, white
water, the very best beverage

## Fast food
light menu items, grilled chicken sandwiches, wraps, salads, real food subs or sandwiches


## The Inconsistent Appetite

The amount of real food that you eat will vary considerably during your recovery. Remember, you may have a stronger appetite at the beginning, to make up for the last famine you were on. Once securely off the feast or famine cycle, your appetite should diminish, or you will be able to tolerate eating less food, so you will eat less. If you know you are off the cycle and your appetite doesn't diminish, you need to guide it along by eating lighter portions and ramping up your quality food intake. Just make sure you stay free of the symptoms of the feast or famine cycle.

## The Guidelines

There's a very simple way to figure out what foods to eat to get variety and balance in your diet: Focus on getting *at least* 8 servings of fruits and/or vegetables a day, literally as much as you want, the more the better. Eating enough of these high nutrient foods is a challenge for almost everyone. If it is for you, work on it. Next, try to get some protein food in with each meal; cheese, poultry or fish or meat prepared simply; or eggs, beans, nuts, seeds, tofu, etc. Don't leave out important starches including potatoes, whole grain pasta, rice, quinoa, other old world grains etc. Quality fats will find their way into your diet through preparation, dressings and condiments. Educate yourself on the best sources.

Always pay attention as you are eating. You may be surprised at how little, or how much you want or need to eat at a particular time. Don't get locked into habit, history, or rigid expectations. Cereal, bread, rolls, crackers, etc. tend to be convenient habit foods. Reserve these foods for times you specifically crave them and avoid building meals around them. Think out of the breadbox here. Some types of beef, lamb, and pork meats are protein rich like fish, although they may be more fatty. Simply prepared, these protein staples are good—but not for every day. Dairy products—eggs, yogurt, cottage cheese, milk, non-dairy milk, etc. are important sources of protein and many other nutrients (and allergens as well).

## Who's In Charge Here Anyway?

Rules about portions here are missing. This places a big responsibility on anyone who decides to apply these principles. There are no strict limits on how much you should eat. All the decisions are up to you. You must figure out what level of quality and what amounts of food will work for you to ensure that you get off the feast or famine cycle. Your job is to avoid getting back into a war with your body by responding to its need for the optimal amount of high quality food all day long every day. Can everybody do this? No. Can you do this? You decide.

This is a big challenge, to be sure. The food avoidant thinking that goes with a lifetime of dieting will probably take a while to conquer. Even after getting off the feast or famine cycle and witnessing all the changes your body goes through, you may easily slip back into faulty thinking. Here's a typical slip that a person in recovery had six months into her enlightenment about food and eating: As her day at the office wound down, Pamela found herself thinking about the date she was going on that night. It's 4:15 and she is hungry, as usual. She thinks, *I ate a good lunch, and we're going out to dinner at 6, so I'll just have some coffee now because if I eat now it will spoil my appetite and I won't be able to enjoy my dinner. Besides, men don't like women who pick at their food.*

Even for a person off the feast or famine cycle for a while, this is a set up for excessive hunger and over eating. Pamela needs to respect her hunger and eat the bunch of grapes she's brought to the office—something that will hold her until 6:30. We all know food doesn't usually appear on the restaurant table for some time after you head for the restaurant. The temptation to restrict food intake or delay eating for hours is all around us and in our heads from years of faulty thinking. Just because we know better doesn't mean we're not vulnerable.

## Food Allergies

Find out if you have food allergies! Undiagnosed allergies can really cause problems for those seeking recovery. One woman I coached who had been stuck for quite a while discovered she had a gluten allergy. She lost 10 pounds in the four months after she took it out of her diet. The best way to diagnose a food allergy is to take the suspected culprit out of your diet for a week or a month, and see how you feel.

## Artificial Sugar and Artificial Nutrients

These ingredients have been staples of dieters for decades because they don't have calories. But saccharine and other sugar substitutes have controversial reputations. Some studies report that artificial sweeteners are damaging to health, causing cancer and other maladies. Other studies suggest that there is no risk to using these sweeteners. The cautionary word here is "artificial." Do we really want to be putting artificial anything into our bodies? That's my position—with the studies that point to potential harm. Recently, there have been reports that even daily multivitamins may also be harmful over time. Mega-doses of specific supplements may also to have deleterious long-term effects. Again, individual responsibility comes into play here. No one can or should decide for you. If you are unsure, do some research.

## Alcohol

I'm putting alcoholic beverages after artificial sugar because there's an artificial food aspect to these pleasure foods, too. Wine, beer and cocktails offer little in the way of nutrients but they do offer significant calories. Just think of this group as you would regular pop—empty calories. I suggest that anyone who does drink and wants to lose weight by learning to eat well on time should either not drink at all or keep their alcohol intake down to one or two drinks a week. And, as always, make sure you have eaten well on the day you choose to drink. Alcoholic beverages can be great make-up foods when people haven't eaten enough, so if you find yourself drinking more than you should, you need to get back to the basics of taking care of your food needs.

## The Fat We Eat

Fat is such a vilified word in diet land that it sometimes evokes anxiety in dieters. But, dietary fat is important! Bodies need it and even overweight bodies need it. (You probably don't believe this.) We have, along with our theories on weight loss, decided that people who have too much body fat must stop eating fat if they are ever going to lose their fat. This is why we have fat-free muffins, low-fat cheese, low-fat milk, no-fat yogurt, fat-burning energy drinks and, if we could manage it, we'd make some product with negative fat! The fat we take out of these foods is supposed to make them healthier and us thinner, but they don't.

The main trouble with taking most or all of the fat out of your diet is that you miss it. Your body misses it, too. It's one of the reasons people go off their diets—they're fat-starved. The only way to prevent this is to keep enough fat in your diet to keep you and your body fat-satisfied. One of the important roles that fat plays in the diet is satiation—a feeling of fullness or satisfaction. Another is the flavor enhancing quality of fat. Although these sound like pleasure issues, they really are biochemical, too. Why do our bodies *miss* fat?

Although fat is concentrated energy—9 calories per gram—it still has a legitimate place in the diet of overweight people. Carbohydrate foods contain 4 calories per gram and protein foods 4 calories per gram, so it would seem logical to eat more from these food categories. And, we generally do. But when fat overpowers the diet, representing the bulk of ingested energy, it's not healthy. Nutrient-rich foods get squeezed out, sometimes even to the point of malnutrition. This happens for overweight people when they get to the feasting part of the feast or famine cycle.

Where does dietary fat fit into this recovery process? The Real Foods list offers some higher-fat foods that are typically forbidden on traditional diets. You are probably thinking, *what are the guidelines here? Can you just drink a bottle of full-fat salad dressing?*

That's precisely the question I wanted you to ask because, of course, you wouldn't drink an entire bottle of salad dressing. So, salad dressings are Real Foods. Now, it is your job to put the salad dressing on the salad, at home and when you eat out. If you want regular dressing, because it generally tastes better than low- or no-fat, put it on as a condiment, not as soup. It's important that you be able to taste the salad. Also, try to get a quality salad dressing made with canola, flaxseed or olive oil. Making your own is probably the best but there are some decent ones at the grocery store, too.

Then, we come to the popular dairy case where almost everything is reduced fat. I was shopping with my tiny, older friend the other day and she reached up for a big carton of half and half. I just had to tell her as a joke, "Nancy, you know, you can get *fat-free half and half!*" She burst out laughing and said, "That's the best oxymoron I've heard in a long time! Kind of defeats the purpose, don't you think?"

But that's where we are when it comes to fat. Well, you might protest, dairy fat is *saturated!* Yes it is, and that's why we have to use our judgment and common sense. If you are new at food quality and good fats vs. bad fats, research this topic. The Internet is packed with helpful information on beneficial fats and nutrition in general. There are also some good books that offer guides to quality foods but beware of the ones that recommend counting calories and fat and all that—it's easy to slip back to diet thinking.

How about butter? Have you eaten a stick recently? Butter is a condiment and can be used with discretion. It is saturated fat so there are a couple of reasons to avoid eating a stick. But, you don't have to eat dry toast with your eggs, even though you know eggs have fat in them, too. *Do avoid* margarine! It's usually made with trans-fats. And, have whole eggs instead of eggbeaters—the real ones are better. Choose real food, not food that's been altered or processed in any way. Cheese is an interesting food. It is almost always mostly fat and that's why they make low fat or even no fat cheese, which tastes like rubber, probably because it is rubber. But real cheese is a perfectly good real food as an appetizer or condiment, not a main course. Cheese often shows up on the appetizer menu for a reason. It's something rich to settle down an overdue appetite. Of course, this won't be the case with you—I mean an overdue appetite. If you like cheese, eat it in small chunks because it has high taste satisfaction and you'll never be so hungry you'll need a brick-sized piece.

**BORDERLINE FOOD**

Just add fat and/or sugar to real foods (this often happens in preparation) or take any naturally high fat, or sweet foods and you'll have some borderlines. These foods offer some quality nutrients but also contain a lot of calories that have relatively little nutritional value. For example, the nutritional value of the beef in regular hamburger is pretty good on the protein side, but its high saturated fat content compromises its quality. Borderlines have their appeal mainly in taste satisfaction and are terribly attractive to overly hungry people, which seem to be most Americans and certainly all dieters. Unfortunately for America, borderline foods have found their way to virtually all restaurants as standard fare. Think French fries, American fries, curly fries. One would think a meal just wasn't a meal without fries to accompany it! It's possible to quickly turn a perfectly good real-food meal into a borderline. Just deep fry it or dip it in chocolate. The Minnesota State Fair actually boasts "deep fried ice cream" as one of its popular offerings.

Some cultural foods are borderlines that people get used to eating because of their ethnic or cultural background. This might make avoiding them quite difficult, but it can be done with commitment and effort. Occasional borderline foods in the diet usually don't derail the person determined to get off the feast or famine cycle and lose weight, but if they do, they have to go.

## BORDERLINE FOOD LIST: Here Are the Types of Foods to Avoid

muffins, waffles, pancakes, French toast
deep-fried anything, fried anything
potato chips, nacho chips, any fried snack chips
French fries, curly fries, ranch fries, crazy fries—you get the picture
dumplings, stuffing
restaurant gravies, sauces, etc.
fast foods except those on the real foods list
bacon, sausage, processed meats (salami, bologna)
pudding, custard
presweetened cereals; high sugar, corn syrup sweetened cereals
pizza with heavy cheese and/or meats (sausage, pepperoni, hamburger)
flavored milk
hot chocolate

## PLEASURE FOOD

The pleasure-food category is self-explanatory, or should be. Foods designed for taste satisfaction alone should not play a regular role in anyone's diet. Nobody really "needs" cherry cobbler, for instance, right? Well, remember that some people do, physiologically at least. Same thing goes for all pleasure foods; cake, ice cream, chocolate, to name a few favorites. People in recovery who want to lose weight have to decide whether they are willing to give these foods up to keep their diet quality high enough to lose weight. Some people are not. It's not that pleasure isn't good, and it's not that eating great tasting food isn't a pleasant experience. It's just that overweight people in recovery *need* good quality food and pleasure food just *isn't good enough food* for them. Many overweight and obese people are actually malnourished because of their extremely poor quality diets. In order to improve their nutritional status, they can't afford to take in calories that don't have a good boost of nutrients.

So how does an ex-dieter stay away from these alluring foods when they are almost irresistible at the beginning, before she's gotten completely off the feast or famine cycle? It's not easy for some. The drive to eat these make-up foods is very strong, but minimizing them from the very beginning has one big advantage. Resisting pleasure foods is a valuable skill for recovery. You might as well get started on that one as soon as you can. It's pretty straightforward but requires three things: eat well all day long, stay away from pleasure foods, and if they show up, just say no, thank you.

**PLEASURE FOOD LIST:**

sweet rolls, pastries
cakes, frosting
chocolate anything
candy, candy bars
cookies and bars
fudge
betties, cobblers, strudel, etc.
pies, dessert pastries
many types of granola bars, check the labels! (often they are glorified candy bars)
ice cream, ice milk, sherbet, frozen yogurt

ice cream concoctions, malts, shakes
sweet toppings, ice cream and desert syrups
soda pop, punch, Kool-Aid—all sugar-based drinks
fruit drinks made partly with fruit juice plus added sugar/fructose/
corn syrup

You probably have a few of your own to add. If you're not sure about whether a food fits into the Pleasure, Borderline or Real Food list, just use common sense.

## FOOD SUBCATEGORIES—At the Gas Pump

Food is fuel. We fill up our tank when we eat so we can keep moving. Here's another way to look at food quality.

I have designed a subcategory to further clarify the good/better/best foods to eat in recovery. It's designed to look at food from a different angle. These categories are divided into the types of fuel that energize planes, cars and trucks. Naturally, you want the fuel with the best efficiency and also ecologically sound. This classification system helps the person in recovery choose the best quality foods as much as possible, giving a bit more structure to the foods lists. It's a way to think of food in terms of a hierarchy in the same way we think of putting gas in our cars. This system can help those in recovery stay with the highest nutrient and overall quality foods.

## Super Octane—All Plant-Based Foods, Fish, Lean Poultry and Meats, Tofu, Dairy Foods

Super-octane foods are pure and efficient and you can **eat as much as you like whenever you are hungry.** Focus on plant-based foods that are generally high in fiber and water, and very high in nutrient value. This list includes *all fruits,* and *all vegetables, legumes.* Bananas—yes! Avocados—yes! Nuts and seeds—yes! Corn—yes! It has always struck me as odd that diets typically put limits on vegetables. For example, one diet I recently read about limited the dieter to 1/2 cup of broccoli! I found this absurd. Broccoli! You could eat a pound and be none the worse for it. The roughage would probably be good for you!

The higher-protein foods are also great quality and you can feel good about eating them freely throughout the day. These excellent foods are like important turbo-fuel in your diet and it's important to choose well from this category, along with fresh foods. Proteins offer valuable lasting satiety as they are generally metabolized more slowly than the plant-based foods. Building your diet around the structure of the plant foods along with these protein-rich foods will keep your hunger well satisfied so you can concentrate on the other important things going on in your life. Always keeping variety and balance in mind, there are no portion limits.

## High Octane—Whole-Grain Foods: Bread, Rice, Pasta, Cereal

This important category contains nutrient-rich complex carbohydrates that are essential as diet staples for many of the world's cultures. But why are they high octane instead of super? In our culture, it has become easy to substitute grain foods, especially bread, for other high-nutrient food groups, like the super-octane foods above. We seem to have a bun on everything and bread with every meal. This category is here to help you learn balance in your eating habits. High-octane foods are excellent sources of nutrients so definitely integrate them into your diet. They should probably play a lesser role than you have been used to (when you are not dieting), and trying to leave them out altogether, as some diets suggest, tends to backfire.

## Regular—White-Grain Foods (Flour, Rice, Pasta, Crackers), Processed Anything (Foods Modified and With Chemical Additives)

Doesn't "regular" sound next to low grade? People don't usually put regular gas in their cars anymore because the new, more efficient engines require higher, purer types of gas to run efficiently. Regular foods are like that. They will work to fuel your body, but they are not as efficient or clean burning and shouldn't have a regular spot in your diet. This is a broad category, including all white flour products and all processed foods. If your grocery cart just lost half its contents, you're not alone. This category of foods probably accounts for much of the make-up foods that people crave and indulge in after they've been on a diet. It may take some practice to eliminate these foods from your grocery list. And, you may have some objections from members of your family about this change. But, never mind.

## Diesel—Rich, Fatty, Sugary Foods, Pastries, Desserts, Ice Cream, Candy, Chocolate, Cookies, Etc.

Do you ever put diesel fuel into your gas-powered car? Would you ever do that to your car? Never? Diesel fuel will ruin your car's engine in no time at all. It would be an expensive mistake to make—very expensive. But, we do this with our bodies all the time. We fill up with diesel fuel and then pay a high price for our recklessness. Once you are off the feast or famine cycle, diesel fuel will not appeal to you as much as in the past. However, you will still have to make decisions, every single day, so drive up to the super-octane pump to avoid these impure and damaging foods.

## Food Availability: What Have You Got to Eat Right Now?

This topic is so important for recovery that I can't emphasize it enough. The main focus in the last chapter was reestablishing communication with your body regarding your need for food. This can only be helpful if you are able to respond to those signals by eating on time—right when you get hungry. We've talked about the absolute necessity of *getting off* the feast or famine cycle, and *staying off* by eating good food on demand. This gives your body a chance to normalize its appetite, metabolic rate, cravings, focus on food, and energy for physical movement. But, eating on demand requires that you make sure your food source is adequate and high quality. Always remember, you can't eat good food when you're hungry if it's not there.

## When Food Isn't There

The foundation of recovery by these principles is first understanding what happens biochemically, inside our bodies, when we get hungry and we don't eat, or don't eat enough, because we're on a diet. Whether dieting or not, poor food availability is almost always the set-up for going hungry and all the overeating that follows.

As we have learned, lack of adequate food is a foundational survival stress for all organisms. Inadequate water is also a basic survival threat. Did you know that your body retains water when you don't drink enough fluid? This is another survival system. In effect, bodies are designed to retain fluid if there's a fluid famine going on. Physicians instruct patients who retain extra fluid to limit salt and *drink more water*. Does this sound familiar? And yet, the idea of telling people who are retaining excess food (fat) to eat *more* good food at the right time seems totally ridiculous—at first.

## Your Environment

Your first and most important "environment" is between your ears—your brain. Your thinking can create food restriction. This is what dieters do. There may be food all around, but when they avoid eating they actually create an environmental famine of sorts. This is a mind-controlled famine. But your actual environment or surroundings can present a true famine too.

Since obesity is a positive adaptation to *an environment* where food is intermittently restricted, we'd better check out the real environments you find yourself in. This refers to where you are—in your home, at the office, in your car, at the gym, visiting neighbors and relatives, at parties and reunions, camping, hotel rooms, airplanes, busses and taxicabs—wherever you are in the world. The reason I list all these possibilities is because we tend to think of our food supply environment as our kitchen, home and restaurants, maybe a snack room at the office or school. But this is one of the main reasons we don't eat on time. We ignore our hunger because there's nothing to eat, or we think of the environment we're in as inappropriate for eating. So we often go hungry. And, our kids go hungry, too. Well, you can't just eat anywhere, can you?

Actually, you can, with very few limitations. People in recovery do figure out how to have food available wherever, whenever they need to eat. They do this because they realize how important it is in order for them to recover from being overweight and the painful diet lifestyle that goes with it. So, they keep great food in their car, in a drawer or small refrigerator at the office. The glove box in their car isn't really for gloves anyway, so they stash snacks there for emergencies. They discreetly drink a protein shake during a meeting at work or have a half sandwich during a short break. You can get really creative about this when you know how important it is for your body. All this eating is on demand, of course, based on your hunger and fuel-full signals.

## What it Takes

I have confidence in those who earnestly decide to break away from dieting and all its physical and psychological destruction and put these principles to the test. I believe in them. I believe that, as they take all the determination and will power they've used as dieters and apply these strengths to recovery, they will learn to be responsible keepers of their bodies. I believe overweight people have the right to eat like normal human beings without criticism or judgment. I believe some have the patience to wait for their bodies to adjust to the important changes they are making and let go of extra weight. I also believe they have the discipline and intelligence it takes to work with their bodies towards recovery. And, I believe they can stand up to the diet-crazed society we live in and spread the good news that there is a way out.

Some who learn about adaptation principles wonder how I can trust overweight people without putting limits on food. *Won't they just eat and eat*, they wonder. And they are wondering about themselves too. It is hard for most dieters to accept that they have built-in controls for food intake, and that they have the ability to gradually manage their eating downward towards weight loss. So at first, they are actually intimidated by the lack of restrictions. Some are afraid of the freedom, and anxious that they will never be able to learn to eat less food in a sane and safe way.

I have found that those in recovery who do the best, who break away from the diet lifestyle the quickest, who find the rhythm and comfort of recovery fastest, are those who grab hold of these principles and stay focused on their job. They don't look for someone else to lead. They don't hope for dramatic changes in their weight because they know it doesn't work that way. They realize that this new life is simply offered and must be consistently and happily applied over years—in fact for a lifetime. They accept that there is no other way and certainly no better way that lasts.

Although you've learned a lot about putting these principles to work, you probably still have some questions: What *exactly* does recovery look like? How do you go about applying all these principles to your life? What is the most important thing to do? What specific challenges can you expect as you go along? What if you get stuck? What if you go too fast? How long does it take to lose weight? Is there any way to speed it up? Does it work for everybody? And so on.

Chapter 6 is all about all these things and even some questions you haven't thought of yet.

# CHAPTER 6

## Evidence That Demands
a New Approach

The track record of traditional dieting is the inspiration for my work and my books. Although this record is dismal, as we have seen again and again, our culture continues to embrace, support, market and promote dieting on a massive scale. Why? Money drives the diet industry and its product: snake oil. If traditional diets are largely insupportable, except as lucrative products, do we have any real evidence that dieting is actually fraudulent? As we shall see, many studies support the idea that biology plays a much more important role than we previously believed. And in light of some of these studies, let's scrutinize several examples of common misbeliefs and some misplaced efforts involving weight loss that appear on television and in schools.

## Biology—Again

I've already addressed the influence that too little food has on bingeing behavior, as well as the role of biochemicals in causing the five adaptive responses to famine. Here is compelling medical research that documents actual biochemical factors that come into play in dieters' rebound experience.

Nutrition researcher Adam Drenowski, Ph.D. said that weight loss experts have traditionally assumed that people who regain weight after dieting simply slip back into bad eating habits. But, he argued, research has documented that the real reason it's so hard to keep unwanted pounds off is lipoprotein lipase, or LPL. LPL is an enzyme that largely controls how much fat you store, he said.

During dieting, the LPL level initially drops and then it rises. It rises dramatically throughout the diet. Scientists speculate that this rise may be responsible for overeating in post-weight-loss dieters. So it looks like this enzyme may be behind the five survival responses I describe, which include overeating.

Another research study by Dr. John D. Brunzell, showed that when obese people lose weight, they start overproducing LPL, which makes it easier to get fat again. The effect of these elevated enzyme levels is to make weight gain far easier for the formerly obese than it is for people who were never fat in the first place. The study found that the fatter people were to begin with, the higher their lipoprotein lipase levels after they lost weight. It was as though the more weight a person lost, *the more the body fought to regain the weight, on a biological level.* This, I believe, is a function of adaptation and high famine sensitivity.

According to the study, the change in LPL levels results from weight that is lost by traditional eat-less dieting, typically weight lost very fast. The question here is, can weight be lost without this LPL response?

Is it possible to lose weight in a way different from dieting and avoid provoking the increase in LPL levels? And if it were possible, could the LPL levels be kept in check to prevent the rebound weight gain that happens with dieting? The next chapter is all about the exciting answers to these and more key questions.

## Sandra

Sandra describes herself as a 22-year chronic dieter. She weighed 198 at her last doctor's visit and she is 5' 1" tall. Her therapist told her she eats to comfort herself because her mother abandoned her when she was 4 years old. Sandra admits she eats "comfort food" when she is alone at night. Although she is convinced that her eating is emotional, what else could be influencing her nighttime over-eating? Could LPL play a role here? Her diet history certainly points to the likelihood that she has elevated LPL levels whenever she diets because she has rebounded literally dozens of times. She must be losing some weight some of the time, but according to this research, the heavier she gets, the higher the LPL levels get and the more likely she is to regain the weight she lost. Is this "comfort eating" or is she in a biological LPL war with her body?

## Make-up Comfort Food

Like Sandra, almost everyone accepts that people eat and overeat for comfort. This idea is related to the "emotional eating" theory. Although we've debunked emotional eating, eating for comfort may have some roots in reality. As we know, dieters and people who eat recklessly experience unmet hunger needs. This leads to excess hunger, which is a particular form of pain. Normal hunger is not painful, but rather a simple urge to seek food, but excess hunger is something quite different.

As we've discussed, excess hunger is especially satisfied with rich food, mainly sugar and fat. We call high carb, high fat foods make-up foods and comfort foods fall into this category. The excess hunger that accompanies dieting strongly influences both the amount and the type of food dieters choose and eat when going off their diets. It brings cravings for make-up food, i.e. comfort food. And why does this particular type of food comfort people so much? Because when extra hungry dieters eat comfort food, *they experience a great relief or comfort—physical and emotional.* The comfort is about their excess hunger, not about the food itself. Of course eating make-up comfort foods comforts them—they are starving and very much need the ingredients in comfort foods! It's really just biology.

Is Sarah a comfort-eater? Is she using food to assuage the trauma of her childhood loss? Does her aberrant eating really boil down to her psychological history? What do you think now? Let's look at a study that suggests that Sarah's past may not really explain her eating behavior.

## Do Overweight and Obese People Have More Emotional Problems than Others?

Thomas Wadden, Ph.D., and Albert J. Stunkard, M.D., did a study on psychological and social problems in obese people. They determined that, although obese people are discriminated against in both academic and work situations,

> ***over weight persons in the general population show no greater psychological disturbance than do non-obese persons.***

They note that although early studies viewed emotional disturbances as causes of obesity, *new findings show* that these disturbances are more likely to be the *consequences of obesity*. The social prejudice and discrimination directed at overweight persons *and the effects of dieting* more likely lead to the disturbances.

The notion that overweight people overeat because they have emotional problems is very popular. The news media promotes this idea and television shows promote it too. This belief is so commonplace that uneducated people and professionals alike readily accept it. But as this study shows, there is no evidence backed by research that overweight people are any more emotionally unbalanced than people of normal weight. We have demonstrated that the coincidental occurrence between overeating, eating comfort foods and emotional distress is not a cause/effect relationship. Rather, these behaviors are linked to the feast or famine cycle.

The theories linking people's emotions and stress to their overeating simply reflect the general state of confusion about weight problems and disturbed eating patterns. There must be some kind of power behind such self-destructive behavior as bingeing on fat-producing foods when you are already 100 pounds overweight! Why would anyone eat so recklessly with their doctor warning them that they are liable to have a heart attack or stroke if they don't stay on their diet and lose weight? What can possibly account for behavior like this? Of course it *appears* that emotions come into play. Emotions are powerful and can cause a whole host of problems in people. I suppose this is why the connection appears so tenable. Even professionals—psychiatrists, psychologists, medical doctors and specialists, obesity experts, etc. cite emotions, stress, and poor self esteem to explain overeating and bingeing, even though research does not support these connections. Actually, the field of obesity research is one of the most perplexing in medical history. Physicians are confused. Obesity researchers are confused and searching for explanations en masse. And a growing number of these professionals are overweight themselves.

Here's another point to ponder. In 1960, the rate of obesity was about 12 percent in our country. By 2000, it was 25 percent. It is now about 35 percent and climbing. The obesity in our country is obvious—just walk down a city sidewalk or stand in line for a movie. Now is it plausible that, in the space of 50 years, human beings have developed such amazing and unique emotional problems, which drive them to overeat and binge, that the rate of obesity in this country has tripled? I don't think so.

## WWI and WWII

We survived two world wars during the 20th century. Surely, war wreaks emotional havoc on all people involved: soldiers, mothers, fathers, wives, and children. In fact, war is probably the most stressful experience humans can endure. If the emotional overeating idea were really true, wouldn't there have been a sharp spike in the number of obese people during and following these conflicts? But, there was not. Well, you may say, by the time the Korean War and the Vietnam War came along, the obesity statistics were starting to climb. Yes they were, and so were dieting and the upsurge in fast food and junk food.

## But...

Let's say that emotions really do cause overeating. What would it take to bypass the alleged emotional trigger to overeat? Since you can't take the emotions out of human beings, can you train people in weight-loss techniques so they don't experience rebound even when they get emotional? What would happen if you trained emotional people to think about food, choose food, measure food, and managing food differently—trumping emotional triggers? Research psychologists call these techniques "Behavior Modification." Do these skills make the difference in people's long-term weight loss success?

In one of his research papers, one prominent obesity researcher expressed his strong opinion about the emotional dysfunction of overweight people. He asserts complete confidence that behavior modification is the crucial link to dieting success. He boldly states: "Behavior modification is the key to a successful program. The diet is only the "bait" to get the patient to modify his behavior. Most obese patients have used food for something other than its basic purpose—i.e. to sustain life. For most of them, food is emotional aspirin; it represents love. It is a way to deal with frustration. It is used for something it was never intended to be. Thus, the critical issue is changing the patient's perception of food by behavior modification."

All right, then. Let's see what this landmark study says.

**Behavior Modification**

Celebrated obesity researcher, Dr. Thomas Wadden, a along with three other prominent researchers, actually put this idea to the test. They set out to improve long-term weight loss maintenance associated with dieting. They divided a large group of patients into three groups. They instructed one of the three groups in behavioral methods of weight control and then compared the outcomes of the three groups. They, too, suspected that behavior modification would make a difference in weight-loss maintenance success.

Here's what they found:

The one-year results appeared to show the benefits of behavior therapy.

**By the five-year follow-up, *"there was not even a hint of the effectiveness of behavioral treatment."***

On average, the conclusions state, subjects in all three groups had regained all of their weight loss at five years and *55 percent of subjects had enrolled in new weight reduction programs.* Famine—feast—famine—feast.

If weight rebound isn't affected by behavior modification, and it isn't caused by emotions or food addiction, then it must be caused by something even stronger—smarter than our heads, more powerful than our will. And it is.

### Professional Prejudice—Ignoring the Evidence

In light of the numerous studies on both LPL and behavior modification, which clearly point to biology and not psychology, it is interesting to find the tremendous amount of prejudice against the overweight among some obesity researchers. I am disinclined to name the researchers I will quote here because their positions are so offensive, unfounded, and even embarrassing. The standard approach these researchers take is a very low calorie diet (VLCD), with very rapid weight loss.

In an offering of maintenance strategies, one scientist implied that overweight people use exercise to "buy calories for fun." Many dieters actually do use this approach, but for *fun?* Tricks he mentions are; unscrewing the light bulb in the refrigerator, storing leftovers in opaque dishes, using a two-pronged fork or a baby's spoon, or substituting some other activity for eating when the urge strikes. The message is clear: avoid food, avoid eating and try to trick yourself into going hungry every chance you can. Even beyond these ideas, he says that patients should throw away their large-sized clothing as part of their psychological commitment to weight reduction. (I wonder what they should wear in the meantime.) He says overweight people must understand that a diet and weight loss will not solve their underlying problems. (Are they *trying* to solve their underlying problems? I thought they were trying to lose weight.) He believes eating is a coping mechanism, and so they must find *new resources and insights* to deal with their lives. They may require psychiatric assistance, he comments.

He continues to assert that behavior modification will make all the difference in long term maintenance of weight loss. This involves psychological support with teaching in methods to keep food intake limited, and weight loss maintained. He asserts that obesity is an incurable chronic disease. (I do not believe this.) And then he states flatly that without treatment, the patient will relapse.

The fact is, *with* this treatment the patient will relapse. Biology trumps therapy and behavior modification every time. Nothing trumps survival. I hope this researcher never develops a weight problem. On the other hand, maybe I hope he does.

## The Bear Facts

The bear exhibit at the zoo offers a unique view or adaptation in these large mammals. It is an enlightening experience. Naturally, I am particularly interested in the description of hibernation because hibernation is a perfect example of a prolonged and extreme famine. How do bears adapt to this threatening environment, completely devoid of food—and water?

The bear exhibit featured a reproduction of a bear den with a brown bear curled up inside and snow thickly packed on top. The exhibit offered a complete explanation of this phenomenon right next to it.

This is what it said: During the fall months, grizzlies and black bears prepare for hibernation [famine] with a bout of frenzied feeding or hyperphagia. They might feed for up to 20 hours and consume 20,000 calories a day—about five times their normal intake! They become very fat, but they have consumed, *almost to the calorie*, the amount of energy they need [to survive] during hibernation. The fattest bears hibernate first. The thinner bears continue to eat if food is available.

What's going on during hyperphagia? It is simply excess eating for the purpose of fat storage as preparation for hibernation. It's actually a protracted binge. How does it happen? Why does it happen?

Bears in distinct seasonal climates hibernate annually, during the winter months. This experience is established from birth. These are the conditions of hibernation:

- no external food or water intake (severe famine)
- dramatic drop in metabolic rate (adaptation to famine)
- no physical output whatsoever (adaptation to famine)

The perfect famine state is accompanied by a perfect drop in metabolic rate to the lowest possible level to maintain life. Bears go into a deep sleep, which allows for near metabolic and physiological stasis. This state is maintained until spring when famished bears leave their dens and seek food again. This spring eating and regaining of weight gradually culminates in the *hyperphasia of autumn when they again prepare for hibernation.* And so, the cycle goes.

Do bears exhibit adaptive cyclical obesity similar to the feast or famine cycle?

## Energy Balance is a Physiologically Controlled Process

A study by Stephen O'Rahilly and I. Sadaf Farooqi reflects this possibility. They say, "obesity *(in humans)* is a *heritable neurobehavioral* disorder that is *highly sensitive to environmental conditions.*"

Dieting, undereating, starvation, excess food availability, inadequate quality food availability, etc. are the *environmental conditions* we're talking about here.

O'Rahilly and Farooqi go on to observe, "Energy balance is a physiologically controlled process. If genetic variation influences body fat stores, then it must do so through biological and not 'metaphysical' [abstract] processes. A body of work stretching over nearly 70 years has clearly demonstrated that energy balance in *mammals* is a homeostatically [equilibrium-regulated] process involving a dialogue between the sites of long-term energy stores, i.e., *adipose tissue*, and the *brain*, which is the organ that coordinates food intake and related behaviors and is the central control of energy expenditure."

So, these scientists have concluded that energy balance in bears as well as humans, both mammals, is biochemically (internally) controlled. Therefore, the overeating, fat storage and use of fat during the feast or famine cycle and the hibernation cycle is a function of biology—and not caused by food addiction or other emotional or psychological problems. Bears and people overeat because they need to overeat. Their survival depends on it.

**But Bears Aren't People**

You're probably wondering if this bears illustration is really relevant. People are much more complicated than bears so you can't really make a valid comparison, right? Human beings experience a whole gamut of influences that animals clearly don't. So, doesn't it seem logical that people with weight problems would struggle with a lot of things that bears don't? Of courses they do. But going back to physiology, underneath all these differences, humans have profound things in common with other mammals. Regarding food, bears and people have similar physiological sensitivities to the environmental food supply, and the same drive to survive—basically the same adaptive potential in this vital area. This is how those two things translate into what we have in common with bears:

- Bears and humans use up stored fat when food is scarce or unavailable. Hibernation and diets are both forms of food scarcity or unavailability.
- Bears and humans eventually overeat and store fat with the cyclic abundant food supply. This is expressed in hyperphasia in bears and rebound overeating in dieters.
- Both bears and humans again use up fat that has been stored when once more food becomes scarce. This is the next cycle of hibernation in bears and the next diet for dieters.

This feast or famine pattern reflects a yearly hibernation famine for bears and a periodic diet cycle for people—sometimes it's a year, sometimes a few months. Bears experience famine yearly and dieters endure famines as long as they can tolerate the food restriction.

The connection between lipoprotein lipase, research on the psychological make up of overweight people, the behavior modification studies and post-diet weight rebound, point strongly in the direction of physiology to explain weight problems. In fact, some obesity research is beginning to go in the direction of physiology rather than psychology. But, the superstitions about fat and weight gain and obesity are rampant. There is still so much uncertainty about obesity even though we have a great deal of evidence that we are barking up the wrong tree. It seems that we only get more confused as new ideas come along. I interviewed the head of an obesity research department at a university and I shared my observation that there is a link between dieting and weight rebound. He laughed and said, "You actually think dieting has something to do with over eating?" I said I did. He laughed again. He was quite fat.

**Rats!**

Studies on rats have yielded interesting results. Dr. Clarence Cohn tested 1,500 young laboratory rats and divided them into two groups. One group was fed at "meal times" twice a day and the other allowed to eat whenever they wanted. The total amounts of food and nutrients consumed were the same for both groups. After 41 days, both groups had gained the same amount of weight, but *the meal eaters had put on almost twice as much body fat.* Other studies have replicated these findings, although in some cases there was a higher food consumption and overall weight gain in "meal eaters" groups as opposed to rats allowed to eat at any time.

What shall we say about rats? Are they troubled in their eating behavior by stress and emotional issues? It seems pretty clear that mammals, in general, are under similar influences regarding their need for and maintenance of extra fat, and it appears that *eating patterns* are very close to the root of this need. The grazing rats were in control of their food intake and the mealtime rats weren't. The grazing rats didn't need to store extra fat because they had a continuous supply of food and ate based on their body signals. Of course, rats are fed only high quality rat food. Right.

If overweight people can't really control the force of adaptation, are they just victims? Do they have no responsibility for their bodies, for their eating, for how fat they are? Is the prejudice against overweight and obese people ever justified? Two of my friends argue that the fat people they know just eat a whole lot of food, and really bad food. Are some people overweight because they just don't care? Yes. Do they deserve to be fat, more than the ignorant yo-yo dieters who keep trying, over and over again to lose weight? Maybe. Is it possible to tell the difference, on the surface, between these two groups of people? No. They are all fat and no one but they know whether or not they are really trying. I personally think most people are trying, at least some of the time. Otherwise there wouldn't be so many people with such serious weight problems.

## How We See Fat in America

In light of the irrefutable evidence that obesity is definitely in part a function of biology, and humans are not on a level playing field where weight problems are concerned, here is a most disturbing study. Thomas Wadden Ph.D. and Albert J. Stunkard, M.D. found "regardless of age, sex race, or socioeconomic status, children as young as 6 describe silhouettes of an obese child as 'lazy,' 'dirty,' 'stupid,' 'ugly,' 'cheats,' and 'liars.' When shown black-and-white line drawings of a child of normal weight, an obese child, and children with various handicaps, including missing hands and facial disfigurement, children and adults rate the obese child as the least likable. This prejudice is relatively uniform among blacks and whites and persons from rural and urban settings, and it is also seen among obese persons themselves."

Physicians surveyed by researchers Maddox and Liederman described their obese patients as "weak-willed, ugly, and awkward." Another researcher suggested that physicians have a prejudice against obese patients because they believe that the overweight are self-indulgent and "hence at least faintly immoral." And yet another scientist looking into this prejudice among health professionals suggests that being overweight is regarded not only as sin, and at odds with the Protestant ethic of self-denial and impulse control, but also a crime for which the person is held responsible. Beyond these moral and legal transgressions, obesity is seen as an aesthetic crime: it is ugly.

And yet, as we have said again and again, overweight people do not have any more psychopathology than people of normal weight! What a resilient bunch of people. This is the shocking irony: There is a clear biological component in obesity which points to some serious forces beyond the control of overweight people. This fact is coupled with a pervasive rejection of the obese as people guilty of the worst of human traits, when many if not most of them are trying hard to solve the very problem for which they are judged.

## Hard to Imagine

Some people maintain their desirable weight by controlled eating. They do not go hungry in general; they do not diet in the traditional sense. They do pay attention to quality in their food choices without ever falling prey to the feast or famine cycle. Often, these people have low famine sensitivity.

It may be more difficult for those who have never dieted, never struggled with eating or with excess weight, to understand the trap of traditional dieting and the no-win struggle that goes with it. In fact, at times I have witnessed judgment and arrogance on the part of some people in this group because they still believe, along with many professionals, that weight problems are a simple matter of self-control and discipline. They can't imagine what it would be like to be in an impossible war with your own body. They have never been in this war, and the biological explanation for excess weight seems like just another excuse to them. We know it's not.

Is it possible to approach this issue in a new way, a way that integrates the biological facts and research cited in this book, and truly treats the whole person, taking the weight of judgment and self-recrimination off for good?

**Poverty and Obesity**

It is evident that biology plays a significant role in predisposing people to becoming overweight, but it should be clear by now that lifestyle absolutely counts, as lifestyle includes eating patterns and food choices. But besides dieting, reckless eating habits and famine sensitivity, what other factors contribute to the obesity epidemic? A significant body of scientific evidence links poverty with higher rates of obesity.

The most powerful factor in the development of obesity is the pattern of eating I've described as the feast or famine cycle, coupled with the availability of extremely calorie-dense make up foods. There are a number of reasons for this pattern of under eating and overeating, as we've discussed, and here's another of real significance. A recent study describes a fascinating link between obesity and poverty. Inadequate income may translate to inadequate food, at least some of the time. For poor people, the feast or famine pattern is simply a matter of real fluctuating availability of money and food. You'd think those in poverty with intermittent food shortages would be thinner than people who eat consistently. But, this is not the picture these researchers paint.

An overview of studies concluded: Overweight/obesity in food-insufficient women may be related to a cycle of food sufficiency (i.e. early in the month when food stamps are available) during which caloric intake may be excessive, followed by a short period of [insufficiency] when resources for purchasing food are limited (i.e. the last week of the month when food stamps have been used). Recent research indicates that food insufficiency may be associated with obesity in women. Girls in households receiving SNAP benefits (dietary supplements) had a *reduced risk for obesity*. Girls in food-insufficient households were significantly more likely to be overweight or obese. The researchers interpreted this as a paradox. We have been discussing this "paradox" throughout the book.

A case study was presented in a radio interview. A woman described her challenge to feed her four children on a limited income. Her poverty made her "food-insecure," according to the researchers. The first two weeks of the month, when there was money, the meals were there, too. The children and mother all ate regular meals and were satisfied, even though the food was not the best quality. But when the money ran low and the food became more scant, the mother said, she stopped eating much of anything, sometimes actually fasting in order to have enough for her children. This cycle is a pattern that had gone on for years. You might expect the woman to be underweight from this intermittent lack of food, but in fact, she said she weighed 240 pounds.

Further conclusions of the study stated that food-insecure adults had nearly twice the risk for binge eating than food-secure adults. Also, a study has documented a cycle of deprivation and overeating among food-insecure parents: When a family is able to obtain food, over-consumption at the influx of food occurs, but when there is not enough food, parents, especially mothers, tend to restrict their intake.

Researchers acknowledge that *intermittent under eating may be related to obesity*. They describe it as a paradox, but it is not a contradiction when you look underneath to what food deprivation means to the body. And then, you must look even below that layer to discover that "food-insecurity" is not a phenomenon that only applies to the poor. The affluent, the middle class, the working class, the disabled—every class of human beings are under the influence of the food insecurity of dieting and reckless eating patterns, and the survival principles of adaptation.

## Nurses

Nurses as a group have an obesity rate over 50 percent. How can you possibly explain such a statistic? I'm a nurse and I think I can.

Nurses, especially those who work as hospital nurses at some time in their careers, are caretakers and caregivers. I have worked as a charge nurse in several hospitals and I have witnessed how nurses eat—and don't eat. The needs of patients and demands of managing medical care often come first. For nurses, this means their patients come before their breaks, which they may not have time to take at all. This means their lunch or dinner breaks may not be priorities either. Nurses' stations and conference rooms tend to harbor cakes, donuts and other treats to get them some quick fuel between their duties. Usually, the most afflicted are women. You'd think, with all the missed meals and walking around they do, they'd all be thin, wouldn't you?

## Going for It

You have to admire very overweight people who show a super commitment to working out at the gym. I mean, aren't they amazing? And their bodies are often amazing examples of how far adaptation will go. Think about it. These struggling people often sweat through one, two, even three hours of working out. Most put themselves under very restricted food allowances because they believe they have to lose it fast or they'll never get there. I'm afraid to calculate the calories burned during their regular visits to the gym.

If there's a trainer involved, the super low calorie regimen should never be allowed, but it often is because trainers can be out of touch with reality too. They may want fast results almost as badly as their charge, and push them along the fast weight loss track. Quick, dramatic weight loss is exciting and rewarding. It's a tangible accomplishment—as long as it lasts. So, an ambitious trainer who gets a hold of somebody 80 pounds overweight might see an opportunity for personal pride and an enhanced reputation. I've recently witnessed a reputable fitness club advertising their 90-day program by telling the story of a member who lost 90 pounds in 90 days. People want this.

Here's a question to help you understand the effect of an extreme exercise program on an obese person. Would you need more calories to hike for 5 hours if you weighed 200 pounds or if you weighed 300 pounds? You'd burn considerably more calories if you weighed 300 pounds. Just think of carrying a 100-pound backpack around all day, whatever your weight. That's essentially what such an obese person is doing all the time. So when he goes on an extreme diet, say 1,500 calories a day, he might as well eat less than nothing. This is what enables people on a low-intake, high-output regimen to drop weight so fast. They soon get into the deficit range and trigger their body's survival defenses.

Obese and morbidly obese people usually go on extreme rapid weight-loss programs that are sometimes medically supervised and sometimes not. If medically supervised, these individuals must be very obese in order to qualify. Whether on a medical regimen or just choosing from the many "quack" weight loss programs out there, very overweight people start by restricting their intake to liquids only. Most liquid diets supply 500 calories a day at the beginning. This is inadequate food for even a child in grade school. But, these people are desperate and admit they have tried everything else. Judging from the list of rapid weight-loss programs that are "medically supervised" on the Internet, a strong element in the medical profession is still committed to, and profiting from, the starvation formula. Some in the medical profession are right there to collect the fees for their "support," without any accountability for long-term results. Would the American Medical

Association sanction *any* serious intervention with a documented failure rate of 95 percent?

## Schools for Obese Children

Childhood obesity is a rising epidemic in our country. A number of schools designed to deal with this problem have cropped up in the last decade. These schools target kids who need a standard education as well as training and support for weight loss. Judging from articles about these institutions, it appears that the standard approach for kids is to take off weight quickly by virtue of a low-fat/low-calorie diet and a great deal of exercise. Does this sound familiar? It's extreme weight loss for children!

The author of the diet to which the children are subjected in one of these well-known schools, is a doctor of psychiatric and behavioral science. Isn't this just the guy you want preparing the menus for a bunch of extremely overweight kids—a behaviorist? Recall the landmark study on behavior modification that concluded that it had absolutely no influence on the long-term maintenance of weight lost by dieting. In light of this study and others like it, this doctor's behaviorism and mental/emotional-focused credentials are questionable, to say the least. Is his background really even appropriate when these kids are up against biology, as studies strongly suggest they are?

We've also talked about the professional prejudices regarding overweight/obese people. This appears to be a good example. Once hired by colleagues who believe that behavior modification is the key to success for overweight people, this behaviorist probably figures these kids are emotional bingers, psychologically disturbed, and food-addicted. It sure looks like they are! He is likely to take the view, since this is apparently still all the rage, that these kids need to eat as little as possible and exercise as much as possible and, voila—massive weight loss will result in just a couple of months. So of course, the diet he designs is a starvation diet from any angle.

Here's an example of a "super lo-fat diet" breakfast for a child at this type of school who may be 80 pounds overweight and working out at least two hours a day: 1 cup non-fat yogurt, 1/2 cup blueberries, 1 tsp. sweetener, 1 cup decaf, 1/8 cup nonfat milk. I am not making this up. They are measuring the blueberries! And 1/8 cup skim milk? Really? There are just over 100 calories in this "meal." Don't forget the bolus of exercise that goes with this "feast."

This doctor may get the result he wants and a big round of applause from the medical community, excited as usual, about weight loss with no regard for the long term. Starving kids and forcing heavy exercise will definitely cause weight loss—*fast weight loss that cannot last*. It is physiologically impossible, and it is an amazing wonder to me that, given the abhorrent statistics on weight loss maintenance after dieting, particularly strenuously dieting, that professionals, yes, professionals, are still barking up the wrong tree—and kids are their victims.

One young man, 15 years old, lost 81 pounds in four months. This averages out to *over one-half pound a day!* Given the carefully controlled food intake and exercise regimens, no wonder he lost 81 pounds in such a short time. He said his depression had completely cleared up with this weight loss, and that's understandable. The trouble is, this school is only designed for one semester per student. Then the students go home where their food intake cannot be controlled and their exercise habits are certainly less rigorous. The kids on the website giving testimonials for the school are all very recent weight-loss successes. Of course, they are.

One fascinating comment in a glowing article about one of these schools caught my attention:

### *"Of course it's one thing to lose weight; it's another thing to keep it off."*

I guess we almost forgot about that part. At least they mentioned it in passing. Then the writer went on: The way kids can maintain their weight loss is by having the *right mindset*. I wonder how they came up with that; the right mindset? Has the right mindset ever worked for you?

## The Good Doctor

I corresponded with a well-known obesity specialist for several months. We agreed, and we disagreed. But one thing struck me as quite amazing: There was a "summit" meeting of many professionals in the field of obesity at one of the schools to which I have just referred. One boy there had lost 102 pounds in one semester, about four months. There was great celebration about this "success." It was pointed out that this kid learned to grow his own vegetables and attended a class on nutrition and weight control, i.e. behavior modification. It was also noted that his self-esteem and his social life remarkably improved. Everyone cheered, hugged and slapped one another on the back over this boy's accomplishment.

One nutritionist wrote an enthusiastic article about how this one boy, (who had *just* lost this weight), had conquered his demons and how, if he could do it then everybody else, can too!

I was aghast when I read about this excitement and naiveté. Surely, a professional *in the field* would be familiar with the statistics on post diet rebound! Of course, with the school's 'round-the-clock support, total control of his diet, and an exercise regimen he could not refuse, this child was bound to lose a lot of weight in a hurry. But so what? It doesn't really mean a thing until he has maintained that loss for at least two years—five years meaning a cure—and his chances of doing that are slim to none, if you'll pardon the expression. Long-term maintenance of this weight loss is impossible, if you factor in the incredible speed with which he lost the 100 pounds and his obvious famine sensitivity. Does this forecast make me cynical? Can't I hope for this one young person's success in his terrible struggle?

I am not cynical. I am realistic. I have been a part of the field for over 30 years. Statistics don't lie—they never lied for me.

# PART III

**Hallmarks of Recovery**

# CHAPTER 7

## Making Peace With Your Body

We've spent a lot of time talking about where we've been—endless diets, cycling up and down in weight and mood, feelings of elation followed by discouragement and depression. It seems as if our whole life has been colored by this quest to lose weight, or maintain weight we've lost. And cycle-by-cycle, we've tried to pump ourselves up one more time with one more diet to try again to eat normally and enjoy a healthy, normal weight. We envy those who seem to stay slender effortlessly. We see that they don't eat less food than we do at any given meal. In fact, we *may* eat *less* than they do, something truly annoying, even maddening.

### Getting it Right

By now, you have learned a great deal about your body—how it responds to dieting, why it recovers the weight you lost on a diet, where your cravings for sweets and fatty foods come from, why you can't seem to keep an exercise program going, and what your sluggish metabolic rate is really all about.

Although this information came with some basic instructions, it's important to bring everything together in a specific recovery plan. Why describe it as "recovery?" Recovery is a process of first accepting that you are going down a destructive path. You've been doing this throughout the book. And then you must commit yourself to the steps toward a new path based on your new understanding. After that, you must persistently practice the new principles, choices and attitudes that lead to healing. Healing means literally to make whole. That is the goal of recovery.

## Where to Start?

First, take a look at your entire diet history. This will help you see the pattern of your losses and gains—the feast or famine cycles. Jot down approximately when you dieted, how much you lost and regained. Go through your diet life right up to now. Then, get specific about the last time you actually lost weight. Was it within the last year? Did you gain it back or are you trying to keep from regaining it? The last year or two of dieting is the most important to consider when determining the initial effect of recovery on your weight. Next, list what your most recent diets have been like: how restrictive, how fast you lost weight and how fast you regained. This information will help you understand generally where your body chemistry is—that it may be ready to store fat as a result of the last famines you went through, even after you start eating well. Recent past dieting is likely to affect how your body initially responds to changing your eating patterns.

## Determine Your Famine Sensitivity

Your diet history may be enough to help you make the leap of faith to stop dieting because it is your personal record, the evidence that dieting is a truly hopeless prospect. Next, assess your famine sensitivity. You can generally determine your famine sensitivity by looking at your own and your close relatives' weight problems. Simply look at your diet history, your weight fluctuations, your parents' weight problems and that of other blood relatives. Weight problems in yourself and these family members will indicate your level of famine sensitivity.

Naturally thin people are usually blessed with two gifts. First, their famine sensitivity tends to be low. This means that reckless eating, eating late, eating poor-quality food on the run, missing meals, make-up eating and going hungry usually do not result in significant weight gain. If they do gain, it is temporary. Their bodies are just not that tuned into the food supply—their eating. They don't have to watch their weight. Their bodies are tolerant of irregular food intake and watch their weight for them. The other enviable characteristic they possess is that they often don't tolerate going hungry very well. Many say they just get too uncomfortable and *have to eat*. Well of course, they do—they don't like the pain of going hungry. What a gift! If the rest of us had suffered with their compelling urge to eat under the influence of hunger, we probably wouldn't have gotten fat in the first place.

## What's the Point?

Because famine sensitivity reflects your body's unique innate programming, it will help you to know where you fall on the famine-sensitivity scale. Ex-dieters with HFS (High Famine Sensitivity) understand that their bodies will not tolerate a significant famine experience—any significant famine. These individuals may take longer to lose weight since their bodies' adaptive potential for fat storage is higher than average; their bodies may be slower to adjust to the changes in the food supply. The good news is that all bodies retain adaptive potential throughout life, and these more sensitive bodies will come along with the same encouragement that everyone else must supply. Those with low and moderate famine sensitivity may not have to be so strict about timing. But, unless they take their body signals seriously, and stay off the feast or famine cycle, they will get stuck.

## Going Shopping

Food availability will end up being your diet and your diet (what you eat) will end up shaping your body. Make a list, examining the refrigerator contents and cupboards for foods you need to replace and want to add to improve your diet. Keep your daytime schedule in mind and troubleshoot areas when you could do better. You may not notice trouble spots unless you really think about your day, when you get hungry and where you are at that time. At the grocery store, take time to look at the fresh produce especially. Try some new foods. Buy fruits you like to add to cereal or yogurt. Get a fresh avocado to eat for a snack—something different. Get creative. Almonds, pecans and walnuts are terrific on cereal or in yogurt or in salads or just for snacking. Splurge on these super foods. You're saving money leaving all the lousy food in the store.

Tape this to your refrigerator in big letters:

### *I will eat the foods I have around.*
### *I will not eat foods that are not there.*

This may sound ludicrous on the surface, but it's not. Actually, it's profound. Remember the adage: Never grocery shop when you're hungry. We tend to buy all sorts of poor-quality food when we are hungry and they are all around us in a grocery store. So, make the decision to eat before you go. If you're not hungry before you go, take some excellent food along with you to eat in the grocery store as you shop, just in case.

Before you shop, think about foods to use specifically for meals and/ or snacks. Always keep variety and balance in mind. For example, stir-fried chicken breast (or a substitute) and vegetables goes well with whole grain rice. Chili (may be meatless) and corn bread make a classic combination. Salmon, chicken, shrimp or just a crust of bread can complement a Caesar salad. Use your own recipes (quality improved if necessary) and meal plans, or adopt some simple, easy-to-make meals from recipe books emphasizing quality and ease in preparation. There are a myriad of cookbooks filled with quick fix high quality recipes. Snacks can be really simple: fruits, vegetables, nuts, seeds, leftovers, salads, hard-boiled eggs, and anything you can easily eat on the go.

## Keep Meals as Simple as Possible

It's a big plus if you are a cook or have one living with you. Here are a few simple ways to get quality, balanced meals every day: If your cook is not at home during the day or able to cook after work, try to make multiple quality meals in advance and freeze them. It's almost as time-consuming to cook a whole chicken or six chicken breasts and a bag of whole-grain rice, as it is to cook two chicken breasts and a cup of rice. A pot of soup or stew can be divided and frozen in multiple servings. Try to turn every food you prepare into multiple convenience foods and you'll always have something on hand. Keep washed fruits and vegetables in sight in your refrigerator, ready to add to a meal or eat alone. Washing and cutting fresh fruits and vegetables in bulk generally consumes just a little more time than doing smaller batches. Always buy prewashed greens for building quick meal salads. You probably have some great ideas of your own by now. The point is, make quality meals immediately available so you never have to wait too long or eat lousy food—this single habit will impact your success more than anything else.

Keep in mind that it's easy to build a satisfying meal from vegetables alone or in combination with grains and legumes, like rice and beans.

If this all sounds like too much, simplify it to work in your world. It is estimated that 25 percent of people in the US live as one-person households. For those of you who live alone, try to resist the temptation to frequent fast food restaurants or quick meals with low-nutrient value. It's challenging to eat well when you are the only one eating. Pre-washed greens can be the foundation for a wonderful meal with other vegetables, meat or seafood, or eggs and your favorite dressing. Keep quality canned soups, stews and chili on hand. Ready fruits and vegetables, (fresh, frozen or canned), nuts and juice are perfect while you put a meal together. If at all possible, learn to prepare simple meals using a variety of foods from the Real Food List. Fresh sandwich shops provide good quality ingredients and are very convenient. Frozen meals aren't necessarily the best quality, but they are usually better than most fast food. Check out the best-quality ones you like and use these if you have to fill in when you are not quite prepared and need a quick meal.

## Ready, Set, Review Preparing for Hunger Away from Home

It's almost impossible to emphasize the importance of this habit. This is a very real issue for people in general and for all people recovering from the diet lifestyle. What do you take with you that are portable, high quality, and spoil-proof?

Maximize quality portable food in your diet: fruits, vegetables, protein shakes (no sugar), yogurt, cheese, and high-fiber foods like dried fruit. Nuts and seeds are great because they have protein, carbs and fat.

Beware of "granola bars." Often, there's very little granola in them. Read the label! Those made up almost entirely of nuts and seeds and/ or dried fruit are the best kind. Look for the higher-protein, lower-carb bars—they stay with you longer. Keep boiled eggs ready to eat. Prepared tuna and egg salad make good snacks. Leftovers from home or a restaurant are good for snacks or meals in a hurry. Fruit, yogurt or almond milk can take the edge off extra hunger while you fix a meal or have plans to eat out.

Many of my clients carry coolers with them so they can have a greater variety of fill-in foods away from home. The advantage to this is that it opens up options for greater variety and changing food interests. And it's usually more appealing to eat fruit or vegetables that have been kept chilled, right?

## Emergency!

But what happens if hunger strikes and you aren't prepared? You're very hungry and in your car. The fast food restaurants are only minutes away. The gas stations with snacks are too. This decision is easy— almonds and a water from the gas station. The nuts are a transition food to get you to real food at home, not a meal, so don't inhale the entire bag. Although it's time for a meal based on your normal schedule, this decision is about preventing you from becoming over hungry and then over eating. Let this situation be a lesson for you in the future.

If you're due for a meal (you'll develop a regular meal pattern as you go along), and can't get to a meal within about an hour, all you know for sure is that you want to find decent food ASAP. If you can find a fast-food restaurant, order the best food on the menu. There are some decent choices at most of the big fast-food chains. You won't be starving if you have eaten well up to this point in the day. Your hunger will be manageable. You can choose well. A salad with chicken, or a wrap should do it. Or get a sub full of vegetables and lean meat. Skip the fries, skip the chips, and skip onion rings, because you *can—because you don't need them anymore.*

## Packing and Paying Attention—Cheryl

When Cheryl decided to start her recovery, she actually took notes the first few weeks, recording the times she got hungry, what types of foods she tended to want and how much, generally. She used the list as a guideline for taking food with her to work. As she went along the first months, she ate the same foods and same portions almost every day. After a few months, Cheryl was confused. She felt disconnected from her body and wasn't getting anywhere. Her diet was high quality, but pretty boring. When we looked at the pattern that had developed, Cheryl discovered that she was experiencing "automatic eating," which is the brainless, habitual eating that ignores body signals. Cheryl was trying to ignore her body signals and eat from memory, in a way. Bodies get used to and tolerate more food than they need if we don't give them some help.

When Cheryl fine-tuned her attention skills and eliminated her automatic eating, she noticed a shift in her ability to get along on less food. Her body was willing but she wasn't giving it a chance to tolerate eating less. When she realized this, she consciously stopped eating just before she felt a clear full signal. She didn't develop cycle symptoms. Cheryl knew this shift wasn't etched in stone—she stayed sensitive to the fluctuations in her appetite—but gradually decreased her food intake, careful to avoid symptoms of the feast or famine cycle. Cheryl lost 60 pounds nine years ago and her weight has gradually decreased since then.

You might find that you need a considerable amount of "traveling" food. This depends, of course, on your work or home environment, your physical activity (the more exercise you get, the more often you are likely to be hungry), your ability to fit meals and snacks into your normal environment, etc. Try packing more good food than you think you'll need just to be safe. During the first few weeks of recovery, you will probably be surprised at the number of times you find yourself hungry at non-meal times. Gradually, you will see a definite pattern emerging in your need for snacks and meals.

Remember to keep quality in mind with all your snacks, but you might find that you need meal food when you get hungry, even when it isn't mealtime. Many people require breakfast when they get up and then another "brunch" in the middle of the morning. These meals keep hunger from soaring at lunchtime, so you're able to make good choices then and stop when you're first feeling satisfied.

Note that it is not unusual to feel hungry when you need to drink water. Always, always keep water with you. Try drinking something when you first feel hungry, especially if it has not been long since you last ate—say two or three hours. This will help with two needs; keeping you well hydrated and double-checking that your hunger signals are about needing fuel.

### Starving for Lunch—Penelope

An 18-year-old student, Penelope had always tried to get through the morning on a diet coke and a piece of toast for breakfast. She was constantly trying to lose 10 or 12 pounds. She thought her trouble was lunch. She was so ravenous by lunchtime that she actually felt shaky until she ate, and often she overate. When she learned about the feast or famine cycle, she recognized this pattern. She started out with cereal at first and graduated to eggs and toast for breakfast. As she learned to pay attention to her hunger signals, she discovered that she was often hungry by about 11. She ate grapes and nuts at 11 and felt comfortable until lunch at 12:30. Her lunches diminished considerably and she enjoyed feeling much more relaxed in the late morning for the first time in a long time.

This small adjustment, along with a couple of bananas or a big bowl of strawberries or pineapple in the middle of the afternoon, transformed Penelope's eating behavior. Her lunchtime overeating disappeared and she actually started to prepare a meal in the evening for herself without the nagging hunger pangs from a day of reckless eating. Penelope didn't have that much weight to lose, and she didn't lose all of it. Her goal weight was too low for her, according to the BMI charts. But Penelope didn't care. She gradually lost six pounds and was so grateful to be able to eat and feel good. That was seven years ago. The part that just baffles her is how she could possibly have lived three years unhappily stuck and miserable, trying to eat less.

## New Patterns Emerge

New patterns of eating develop for those applying these recovery principles. Again, it is common for these individuals to eat twice before lunch, then lunch and again mid-to late afternoon before dinner (or supper), ending the eating day with dinner. It's best to have supper on the early side, based on your hunger, and to be done with eating until the next morning, unless you need a snack in order to sleep. People who exercise in the evening are likely to need a snack sometime before bed. Examples of good evening snacks are fruit, juice or any type of milk—bananas are particularly good for this.

You may ask, *why is it OK to go hungry after supper? Isn't this a famine?* If you've eaten well and enough during the day, the empty feeling you have before sleeping is a good signal that your body can rest from digestion during the night. If you are still overeating or needing to eat a meal at night, this means you are still on the feast or famine cycle and you need to boost your eating quality food on time during the day. After supper, eating anything but a small snack will not only force your body to work to digest this food while you sleep, but it also sends the signal to store fat. Studies show that people who eat most of their calories during the earlier hours of the day tend to maintain or lose weight whereas those who eat the majority of their calories later in the day tend to gain weight.

So it's *beneficial* to go to bed hungry. In fact it's a good goal. The ability to comfortably avoid eating food after supper is one hallmark signal that you are off the feast or famine cycle.

## Habits Can be Confusing at First—Glenda

It took Glenda quite a while to get the hang of eating on time and having enough good food around to eat when she got hungry. Working as a veterinarian assistant and attending college, Glenda had some significant schedule obstacles to work through. At first, she kept trying to gauge her eating by the clock—a habit she'd had for many years. So, tuning in to her hunger as the primary "eat" signal was her first hurdle. It took a while. Then, Glenda had trouble with eating mid-morning, even though she discovered that she was hungry an hour or two before lunch. It just didn't seem "right" having two meals before lunch, plus it was nearly impossible to fit in two meals in the morning. She took food to eat for this trouble spot and behold, her lunches got smaller and her nighttime hunger signals quieted down. By this time, she felt she was on her way, although the problem of food availability was still an issue.

Glenda was so used to avoiding food that she said the idea of actually bringing it with her was pretty weird. At first, she just figured she'd use the vending machines at work to get snack foods when the urge struck. But after a few weeks of this method, Glenda knew her food quality wasn't so hot. She decided to actually shop for some decent snacks and have them with her in her car, her desk at the office, and in her gym locker. This shift made all the difference. Not only was it more convenient, but also the quality of her overall diet improved significantly.

There was one other problem Glenda had to solve: how much to eat "between meals." Glenda had been on many diet programs and was programmed to eat, say, 10 almonds, as a snack. That was the limit. It had nothing to do with her hunger satisfaction but with calorie control. We discussed this and Glenda decided the only way to break her habit of "medicating" her hunger instead of satisfying it was to consider each experience of hunger that was more than about three hours after the last meal as a "meal-level" hunger. Medicating hunger is eating when you're hungry but limiting the amount so you just take the edge off your hunger. Sometimes you may need a meal followed by a meal and then a snack followed by a snack. Don't get rigid about how much to eat when. When you are meal-hungry, medicating that hunger with a snack can leave you hungry again soon after.

Glenda had an up-and-down experience in her recovery but she persisted because of the dramatic changes in sensing her hunger and fullness. She had never really felt full before, as far as she could remember. Glenda wasn't perfect in applying the principles but she lost 25 pounds six years ago and gained the freedom to eat and satisfy her hunger all day, every day. She does wrestle with food availability from time to time, and has to keep working on that, but now she knows what to do if she gets off track; just get back to basics. She has maintained her original weight loss, with small fluctuations, for nine years.

There are situations where "medicating hunger" is appropriate. For example, when you are very close to eating a meal and you find yourself quite hungry, have something light to keep yourself from becoming over hungry. Fruit, vegetables, nuts, or some cheese and crackers are fine. This will help you to eat moderately at the meal. Never let yourself get to the starving point. Also, as you move through the stages of recovery, you may experiment with satisfying your hunger by eating less food than you are accustomed to eating. This is a form of medicating your hunger. When it is ready, your body will tolerate a lower food intake to accommodate weight loss. As long as you don't develop cycle symptoms, this is the way to support your body in using up excess fat and achieving your best weight.

**The Goals Before the Ultimate Goal**

In order to get thin for good, **your primary goal is to get off the feast or famine cycle.**

If you don't get off the cycle, you may lose weight but it won't last. Remember, it's the cycle of famine followed by feasting that triggers the body's need to store excess fat. So if you don't break this cycle by consistently eating well (and only you can determine *how well*), your body will continue to be programmed to store fat as famine insurance.

But what if you get off the feast or famine cycle and then get back on again? **Your secondary goal is to stay off the feast or famine cycle.** You must stay off the cycle consistently or your body will return to the pattern of the yo-yo diet cycle and the biochemicals that cause weight rebound.

Does this mean that you will be practicing these recovery principles for the rest of your life if you want to stay thin? Yes. Is this realistic? Yes.

**Symptoms of the Feast-or-Famine Cycle:**

**Here's a simple checklist to keep you aware of the trouble signs of the feast or famine cycle:**

1. Overeating/bingeing (eating until you feel overfull, stuffed)
2. Preoccupation with food and eating
3. Cravings for sweets and/or fatty foods, eating sweets, fatty foods
4. Intermittent low energy, depression
5. Eating without "real hunger," especially at night
6. Eating in response to emotional cues or stress or boredom
7. Special-occasion overeating
8. Excessive hunger or symptoms of low blood sugar (headache, faintness, irritability, anxiety, confusion)

This list will help alert you if your eating behavior is getting off track so you can make corrections to get back on track. Until you become so accustomed to body-controlled eating that that it becomes second nature, it is crucial that you give yourself a regular check-up. Sometimes people go many months with symptoms of the cycle but are not aware of it. Consequently, they get stuck either gaining weight or in a plateau.

**Alice**

A 35-year-old middle school teacher, Alice didn't really believe the adaptation ideas when she first heard them. She had gained 30 pounds during the 10 years after graduating from college. She agreed with the adaptation concepts but the notion of losing weight by eating when she got hungry, even only great food, sounded ludicrous to her. So she kept dieting and she kept losing and she kept gaining it back. When she reached her top weight, 38 extra pounds, she decided that maybe dieting wasn't the answer for her after all.

Alice figured her famine sensitivity was moderate and her last diet was over two years before. So she started tuning in to her body for cues to eat and cues to stop. She was doing the best she could but still, nothing happened. For six months, nothing happened. Discouraged and ready to quit, Alice contacted me. I advised her to take a closer look at her new eating patterns, looking for trouble spots. Although she ate a solid breakfast, she was getting too hungry in the middle of the morning and overeating at lunch. As a teacher, it was very difficult to get even a small snack in at that time because she was doing individual meetings with her kids while they were eating snacks. And Alice also found herself shaky while she fixed dinner, trying to hold off for the meal with her husband. She struggled with hunger after dinner every night.

Here are the simple changes Alice made to get back on track: During the midmorning meeting with her kids, Alice decided to eat a snack, too. Why not? This was so practical and easy, she wondered why she didn't think of it before. Getting too hungry before dinner was rather easy to fix, too. She started taking fruit and nuts in her car for her drive home. By the time she got there, she felt much calmer and ready to relax for a few minutes before cooking, without all that discomfort. If her husband was delayed and she was hungry, Alice went ahead and ate without him. Her evening hunger disappeared.

These were two famines Alice experienced almost every day. Once she discovered them, she was able to make adjustments and get on with her recovery. A month later, her eating became a comfortable routine and within six months her clothes were getting noticeably roomier.

**Here's the checklist of signs that you are in recovery, consistently applying the principles:**

1. Clear hunger and fullness signals
2. Intolerance of excess hunger

3.  Boredom/disinterest with eating
4.  Easy ability to avoid pleasure food, borderline food
5.  Plenty of energy, positive outlook
6.  No eating from non-hunger cues
7.  Easily avoids after supper eating
8.  No excess hunger
9.  No make-up eating/overeating
10. Tolerates eating lighter foods/smaller amounts

This is the list you want to describe you, consistently moving along in your recovery. Contrast it with the symptoms of the feast or famine cycle above. As a dieter, that list is an accurate picture of your former war with your body. This new list—symptoms showing you're off the cycle—reflects the experiences that mark a brand-new chapter in your life with your body. Use these lists to check up on yourself, especially at the beginning stage of your recovery, which is quite different for everybody. The best way to tell if you are moving beyond this first stage is your awareness of a rhythm—an ease in your eating pattern. You sense that this way of eating has become second nature to you. You wonder why you ever lived any other way.

**Fear of Famine—Overdoing it**

Many in recovery develop a fear of famines—the least amount of hunger that may go unsatisfied. Recovery is designed to eradicate fear about food and eating, so this is ironic. But it is understandable, too. Since going hungry regularly is the stimulus for fat storage, then anytime you are even a tiny bit hungry and not eating immediately, you might be tempted to think you are you risking tripping the fat storage lever. But once you are off the feast or famine cycle, mild hunger that does not lead to cycle symptoms is a normal part of recovery.

Fear of going hungry is not what this program is all about. After you are securely off the feast or famine cycle, the immediacy of eating is not as crucial, but we have to be careful here. It's easy to get really sloppy and rationalize eating too late and getting into trouble. At rest, once you're off the cycle, it's OK to tolerate *mild* hunger for perhaps 30 or 45 minutes, even an hour. Remember, hunger is not the problem—excessive hunger is the problem. So eating in a way that prevents excessive hunger is the simple goal. Don't panic, just plan. The important thing in these situations is that you are not physically active and the hunger is not too strong. If you don't tolerate going this long and develop symptoms of the feast or famine cycle, close the hunger/eat gap.

Remember, you are learning how to eat like naturally thin people. As I mentioned, the only time to be especially careful about closing in on the hunger/eat connection is when you are physically active.

## Hunger and High Activity

Let's say you are working out on the treadmill and you had cereal or a shake a few hours before. Suddenly you feel hungry—very hungry. What should you do? You'll have water with you so drink some water. When you are finished with your workout and your hunger reappears, have something right away. If your hunger remains strong during your workout, stop and get something light—fruit juice or a small smoothie, and if you have quite a ways to go, have a bit more so you feel energized and satisfied but not full.

## Haley

Haley worked as a legal assistant after her first baby was born. She was 26. She began her recovery after eight years of dieting, including her latest attempt to lose her "baby weight." Haley said she was glad for permission to eat—just that—to be able to eat. As she got off the feast or famine cycle, she noticed she couldn't tolerate going hungry—at all. This was a big change for her. Her hunger often hit so hard that it was impossible to miss and she learned quickly to keep good food with her. Actually, many of those in recovery report this change. When they were dieting, they were comfortable going hungry, but when they began to eat on time, satisfying their hunger every time it occurred, their bodies began to send strong, undeniable signals.

Haley's challenge was obvious, and she was up to it because of the relief she felt at not having to go hungry anymore. Her strong hunger signals actually made it easier for her to stay on track. She lost 22 pounds, but it was not as much as she had wanted to. This was distressing to her until she weighed in at the doctor who said Haley's BMI was 22, well within the optimal range. Right through a second pregnancy, Haley's been diet-free and fat free for four years.

It is fairly common for women, especially, to have unrealistic weight loss goals for themselves. Often, these women are young and are influenced by the media even more than those older than they. Some hope to get to a weight they were in high school or even junior high. I was one of these women. When I began my recovery, I wanted to weigh 120. I am 5' 8". As I look back, this was obviously an unrealistic weight for me. As I learned to eat and gradually lost weight, I leveled off in the mid-140s. So, I just waited, impatiently, as the scale stood still. It stayed at that weight for almost two years before it dawned on me—that was it. I wasn't going to lose any more. I still wanted to be thinner, but I wasn't willing to fight my body to get thinner. So I accepted my body's decision and, except for a temporary bump up during menopause, I've been right around that weight ever since—33 years.

Some bodies are naturally tolerant of going hungry, which I've described as a problem for weight sensitive people. For example, Chuck got off the cycle and experienced hunger in a rather pleasant, gradual way. Mid-morning, usually at about 10:30, he'd notice an empty feeling and a vague interest in getting something to drink and eat. But he didn't feel compelled by it. Although this subtle message from his body was less urgent, it was just as important for Chuck to learn to respond, knowing it had been three hours since breakfast.

## Traitors in the House

Many people ask me about living in a household where other people are dieting or not committed to eating healthfully. This is a bit of a challenge, but there are tactics that can make it less difficult. The biggest problem I've found for those who share their homes with sloppy eaters is the pervasiveness of poor-quality food. These tempting items may interfere with your recovery, but we live in a real world with really bad food all around us. It's important to get used to avoiding the junk and, if you have the opportunity to practice staying away from it at home, do just that. This is a program of prevention—preventing overeating and eating poor-quality foods—by eating great food consistently. A person in recovery, if she has stayed off the feast or famine cycle, and consistently followed the basics, should have little trouble saying no to borderline and pleasure foods, even if they are in her own home or office. Stay fed-up and you'll be able to just say no.

## Barbara

Barbara weighed 245 when she came for counseling. She was 5'4". She had dieted off and on for 18 years, with a starting weight of 152. When she told her husband, Rod, her plan of never going hungry because going hungry eventually made her gain weight, he laughed at her. She felt hurt but determined. And it seemed as if Rod was determined, too—to derail her efforts. This is an irony of close relationships and

137

it is not uncommon with this program. Family members will insist on bringing potato chips and dip, baked sweets like brownies, ice cream and favorite candies home while the person they say they care about struggles to change something extremely important in her life. It's just too bad. Unfortunately, Barbara was unable to recover. She struggled with eating on time and eating quality foods consistently, partly because her husband actually fought against her efforts to get off the feast or famine cycle.

## How Important is it to Avoid Borderline and Pleasure Foods?

Invariably, my clients who continue to choose borderline and pleasure foods and struggle with cravings for these poor-quality foods are not eating high-quality food on time. They remain on the feast or famine cycle. The avoidance of low-class food is crucial to recovery for the vast majority of people and unless these poor quality foods become very scarce in the diet of a person wanting to lose weight, there's little hope for recovery. If there were an easier way, surely we would have discovered it by now. You simply have to choose.

Are borderline foods ever OK? First of all, if you're interested in losing weight, eating foods with a lot of fat and/or sugar will definitely hold you back. Fat is concentrated calories that doesn't require much energy to maintain or digest, and sugar is non-nutritive and great for building fat. Your goal in recovery is to *optimize* your food quality, which means you minimize the rest. This doesn't mean that you can't *occasionally* have bacon or sausage with your eggs (morning is the best time to eat foods higher in fat) it just means that borderlines are exceptional foods for once in a while. What is once in a while? It's about every two weeks.

## Are You Serious?

They say that if you aim for nothing, that's what you'll hit. Although it is unwise to be too rigid about a specific weight-loss goal in a time frame, keeping your aim steady on great-quality food, eating on time, paying attention to fuel-full signals and exercising at least three or four times a week, is essential to your success. But, it's easy to slack off and become complacent.

I've coached people who are stuck and tell me they're eating fried foods and desserts once or twice a week, because they want to. They figure if they want to then they have the right. And they do. When I ask them about their goal concerning their weight invariably they say they want to lose weight, but what harm can cheating do if they follow all the other "rules?" I'll tell you. Low class foods send your body the wrong message and that message is, "Time to store up for winter." It's certainly fine for people to eat whatever they want whenever they want, but they have to accept their bodies' sensitivity to the food supply. That means having realistic goals.

If you don't really care that much about losing weight, go ahead and eat whatever you like, any time you want. Nobody's saying you can't. This isn't a legalistic program; it's a program that requires the personal responsibility of each individual in recovery. There are no "rules," but only information, guidelines and suggestions. Your food choices will reflect your goal—what you're aiming for. A borderline or pleasure food once in a while should not derail your recovery, but who knows?

## Is Your Goal Realistic?

The desire to be under weight is so common because of our cultural preoccupation with thinness and beauty. It's also one of the things that keeps even thin people dieting—they imagine that they should be even thinner than they are, or they are afraid if they don't keep dieting they will simply gain weight spontaneously. The best approach to avoiding this pitfall is to keep your expectations open. Your body will adapt to the food you supply and to your activity level. Your job is to supply the food and get consistent exercise. The weight you will eventually achieve will reflect these two components. You do your job: Eat the very finest food on time that you possibly can and keep your body moving. If you stick to your job, your body will be able to find your best weight.

This is a program of cooperation between you and your body. You can follow it forever because you and your body are working together toward the same goal—not a number but a lifestyle and a relationship. It's not an archaic method that violates your body's survival instinct, but a sane eating approach that eliminates the bingeing, cravings, overeating, excess hunger, focus on food, anxiety, fatigue and feelings of desperation that go with dieting. I know this is possible for you. It happened to me and it's happened to many others who were willing to take the plunge.

Although you may still be skeptical, *you can* learn to eat like a normal person, learn to integrate more movement in to your life and eventually achieve a normal weight. You already know quite a lot about how to actually do it, but some essential specifics are coming right up!

# CHAPTER 8

## Ending Dieting Forever

Welcome to reality! Most of these principles will be familiar to you by now, but some special information is essential to your success— your lasting success. First of all, remember that what you are going to do requires you to maintain a complete paradigm shift from the traditional diet approach. Food is no longer your enemy—it's your best friend.

Your body is designed to resist anything that brings disequilibrium, which is a state of imbalance, and naturally opposes changes—even beneficial ones. Consequently, when you get securely off the feast or famine cycle, your weight will plateau for a time. This interval is necessary for your body to reestablish equilibrium while it tests the change in the food supply, whether it is temporary or lasting. This plateau period is different for everyone and depends on many variables. Your job is to stay focused on the food supply—the quality and adequacy of food you are eating.

Remember the five adaptive responses to dieting? They are increased appetite, lowered metabolic rate, cravings for sweets and fats, preoccupation with food and eating, and avoidance of physical activity. When the dieting stops, and the pro-active quality eating begins, the body doesn't have to struggle to adapt to limited food any more with these five mechanisms. So, what does it do? Through biochemical changes, these five adaptations reverse.

## Re-Adaptation to a New Food Supply

### 1. Decrease in Appetite

This change doesn't happen all at once, but when it does start to show up, the people who experience it become almost giddy with excitement. They just can't believe that their bodies are capable of doing this amazing thing: They simply do not want as much food. Sometimes, people are so skeptical of this that they try to keep eating the amount of food they're used to, but they get uncomfortable and have to back off. They start eating lighter foods, smaller portions, and leaving food on their plates. The lowered appetite announces a new need in a body; a need to use up excess fat that has become maladaptive in this new environment of an optimal food supply.

Sometimes this shift is not obvious and can be missed. Sometimes bodies resist this change because it is stressful. If you are off the feast or famine cycle for several months and your weight and eating are stable, you can be confident that your body is ready for a fuel reduction in terms of both quality and amount of food. Move toward more plant based foods and/or stop eating just before your fullness signal. You should know your body well enough by now to do this easily. But you must make changes gradually and be sure you don't get back on the cycle. You should tolerate a lowered food intake well if your body is ready for it. If it isn't and you have feast or famine cycle symptoms when you back off on your eating, then wait a week and try again.

Is this lowering food intake just another form of dieting? No. It requires that you first stay off the fat producing cycle as you lower your intake of food. As long as you remain free of cycle symptoms, you know you and your body are not in a war but are working together. You and your body have to cooperate to decrease your overall food intake in order to lose weight for good. Without the chemical influence of a famine, this adaptive change is finally possible!

## 2. Increased Metabolic Rate

A body's conserving energy when fuel is limited is simply logical. So reversing this formula by supplying plenty of high-quality fuel makes sense, too. A depressed metabolism that goes with dieting can cause symptoms of depression, lack of motivation, poor of energy, low body temperature, and weight gain. Maybe you've had some of these symptoms as a dieter. The good news—speeding your metabolic rate up—will happen gradually as you eat better. Eventually, your metabolism will be humming along at its optimal level because your body will be appropriately fueled. Naturally, this shift will contribute to gradual weight loss, and just plain feeling better.

There are two ways to stimulate the metabolism: Everybody knows one of them—exercise! But no one ever talks about the other one: eating! Isn't that wonderful? When you eat, your body has to use up calories to digest food for its energy needs, and that stimulates your metabolic rate. Instead of conserving calories, your well-fed body can afford to waste energy in the form of heat.

## 3. Loss of Interest in Pleasure Foods

Besides clearer body signals, your *appetite* for poor-quality foods—sugary, fatty, processed foods that you used to be drawn to will dwindle. They will start to look much more like what they really are: unappetizing, poor excuses for food. As you consistently eat high-quality foods, your *need* for these make-up foods will wane dramatically. When you were waging a war against your body, cravings for make-up foods were probably a source of anxiety, frustration, guilt, confusion, remorse and shame. You may have associated these cravings with your emotional or psychological inadequacy. But always remember; these cravings are *symptoms*. They aren't symptoms of your defects, but symptoms of your body's attempts to manage your eating patterns to stay alive. Now you can kiss your fat-producing cravings goodbye. It's a wonderful experience to realize these poor quality foods have no power over you anymore.

## 4. Focus on Life

Your attention has been over-focused on food as a dieter because you haven't been getting enough of it consistently while trying to lose weight. Now that you're getting plenty of good food whenever you need it, you can get on with your life and pay attention to other important things, letting your body and your commitment to food quality manage your food intake. It's a wonder how ex-dieters go from preoccupation to nonchalance in their attitude toward food. Aside from making sure there is enough quality food around, those in recovery just don't worry about eating. In fact, it bores them—something some complain about. But they don't complain too much because they say they finally have time, energy, and focus to live their lives, free from obsessing about their eating and their weight. There's more on this significant shift coming up.

## 5. Desire for Physical Activity

With the energy supplied by plenty of great food, and the increase in metabolic rate, your interest in moving around is going to take a leap. Bodies are built to move around, and it's only when we abuse them that this instinct is suppressed. Now that you understand what you've been doing to yourself, you feel better about yourself, and you feel better about your body—even while you are still overweight. And, you feel more like actually doing more physically. You probably never thought it would happen, but it did—or it will. So, go with it! Keep moving around more, teaching your body that it doesn't have to struggle against a lousy food supply anymore. Tell your body you're sorry, that you didn't know, and that you're changing the whole plan, for your body's sake, for your sake, and for goodness sake!

## Review of re-adaptation to the new food supply—reversing the five adaptive responses to the feast or famine cycle:

1. Decrease in appetite
2. Increased metabolic rate
3. Loss of interest in pleasure food
4. Focus on life
5. Desire for physical activity

## New Eating Patterns

The changes in your eating patterns will promote the biochemical changes in your body for the gradual change in your weight. The landmarks below may not occur in order, and will overlap with each other and with the five adaptive reversals above. Sometimes, a step forward will be followed by a step back temporarily. Just look for the momentum aimed generally toward your goals.

You've probably started eating by these recovery principles and you may have already experienced some changes in your hunger, fullness and your eating patterns. You will experience definite shifts in hunger during the first weeks of body-controlled eating, even if you aren't doing it perfectly.

First of all, your body signals are becoming quite definite. You may find that you don't tolerate your hunger as well as you used to. Your body may not be as tolerant about waiting for food once you get hungry. And, you may start realizing that you are hungry for specific foods at times. You should also know when you are full and want to stop. These changes are the hallmark of your body getting the message that the famines have stopped. Even if you don't experience these changes at first, be persistent in eating well, demonstrating to your body that there will be no famines in the future.

## Food Preference Shift to High Quality

This interesting change coincides with the decrease in cravings for fat-producers that recovering dieters experience. As people in recovery become well fed, they become more interested in higher quality foods. This doesn't mean they always want the best food and never yearn for a dessert. But, once the feast or famine cycle is broken, people just tend to *want* better food. Those in recovery find this very interesting and sometimes shocking. They've been trying to stick with decent food on diets for years and couldn't because they were too hungry. And now they want the food they know they need. Finally, they are fighting on the same side as their bodies and this amazing cooperation begins to take place.

## Emotional Changes—Mary

Mary had been so hooked into dieting and trying to avoid eating for so long that the idea of being able to eat whenever she felt the urge seemed like heaven. She dove into her recovery with complete abandon and wrote in her journal about her experience from day to day. The biggest changes for her were emotional. She hadn't realized how pervasive the diet lifestyle had been in her life, and shortly after starting she said she honestly felt like a new person. Even though she'd only been in recovery for a few weeks, her fear of food was gone, her self-esteem improved considerably, she finally felt comfortable eating in front of other people and just felt so much better physically, without the almost chronic hunger she'd suffered for years. She even felt better about her body, although nothing had actually changed—yet. Seven months into her recovery, her clothes were getting a bit looser. Mary considered this weight loss just a bonus to being freed from dieting.

## Eating Shifts to Earlier in the Day

As we've discussed, dieters, and many others, typically eat less food earlier in the day and more in the evening. We know the reasons: they tolerate hunger earlier in the day, their resolve is stronger, and their hunger is not as overpowering. But late in the afternoon and toward suppertime, many dieters struggle to stay in control. This is the time many people "go off" their diets. We understand this too.

But those in recovery, free to eat whenever they get the signal, learn to eat more food early in the day. Because they avoid eating in the evening, they naturally experience greater morning hunger. As a consequence, these ex-dieters develop new eating patterns: breakfast, brunch, lunch, mid-afternoon, and evening. I've talked about this before because it's *very important*. This shift in eating is an essential part of the end of the feast or famine cycle and the beginning of a body's recovery from intermittent famines and the need to store emergency fat. I've noticed that the mid-morning and mid-afternoon snacks or mini-meals are crucial to keeping lunch and dinner high quality and moderate.

## Skill in Navigating the Real Food/Engine Fuel Lists

At first, the Real Food category can be overwhelming—so much food, so few limitations. But those in recovery gradually learn to use this list better as their interest in quality foods grows and their cravings for poor quality food diminish. Most have to learn about what great food, and variety and balance look like. In the diet days, rules about foods on the diet and forbidden foods may have made the choices easier. But the downside of this is that it is not realistic; dieters don't have to make the choices for themselves. Plus, rebound dieters may find forbidden foods particularly irresistible once off the diet. But those in recovery can own their diets, and choosing from the Real Foods list becomes easier to do as they become more experienced and more knowledgeable. They know you can butter your toast, put mayonnaise on a sandwich, and use regular salad dressings, as long as you stay well fed all day long and use your head. Recovery is not a license to eat irresponsibly. It's a plan to eat in a sane and responsible way for your health and your life.

## Getting Used to Balance and Variety

It may seem like a daunting task to integrate more fresh and wholesome foods into your diet, but this is the way people who recover get started and it feels more and more normal as they go along. In time, it's second nature and they look back and wonder how they ever survived the complicated diets they went on. Eating should not be particularly complicated. Eat a variety of foods every time you have a meal and choose snacks to fill in important whole foods you may miss at meals. Select from three or four of the food groups throughout the day, always having fruits and/or vegetables every opportunity. Maybe there are foods you tend to avoid from habit and need to add to your diet. And perhaps you would enjoy learning to prepare new recipes to add variety. There are many resources for quality eating information available on the web and in bookstores. Snack times are great for integrating fresh foods, but be careful here. Very often mid morning and mid afternoon snack time requires something more substantial than a few carrot sticks. A piece of fruit midmorning may not hold you very well until lunch, but that's what you want—you want to spoil yours appetite for lunch so you can eat a quality meal comfortably. So your snack might be two oranges or bananas and nuts, or a bunch of broccoli with dip and a bunch of grapes. You know what I mean.

**Eating Mostly Plants**

I keep saying things like, "Always having fruits or vegetables at every opportunity." With all this talk about focusing on plant-based foods, it sounds like you might as well become a vegetarian. Well, you might. Or you may choose to minimize animal foods, keeping plant-based foods front and center in your diet. The main advantage of staying with all or mostly plant foods is that you are assured of high quality in your eating. Variety will still play a role in your dietary choices but you are certain to be eating good, solid food with high nutrient value.

There are some down sides of vegetarian and vegan eating. The main one is plant foods, in general, may not keep you full as long, and it is easy to become over hungry if you don't plan carefully. This is why people who become vegetarian to lose weight don't lose it—they stay on the feast or famine cycle. So the same principles for getting off the cycle and losing weight apply here. Another consideration about going vegetarian is getting enough plant protein. Bodies need a complete set of amino acids from dietary proteins regularly and animal foods provide this. Vegetarians and vegans have to combine plant foods to form these complete proteins.

If you are headed towards a partial-vegetarian, complete vegetarian or a vegan diet, it's important to educate yourself about this issue.

Am I recommending a plant-focused diet? Yes. A lot of research points to the superior aspects of this type of eating. Does this mean you have to give up meat or dairy to recover and lose weight? No. But I have found in coaching those who are stuck that their recoveries start moving along when they stay off the feast or famine cycle and switch to plant-focused eating.

## Boredom with Food

You've probably snickered about this idea earlier on. It is a real switch and it really happens—it happens to virtually everyone in recovery. They feel hungry and go to the refrigerator but nothing looks appealing. They don't want to eat even when they're hungry! This points to your body's need to pull you back on food intake and it is a clear indication of getting/staying off the feast or famine cycle. You do have to eat less food than you are using up to lose weight, right? Well, this time you're not forcing the change—your body is re-adapting, and you are helping it along: Your appetite goes down, sometimes by your general disinterest in food. All of a sudden, it seems, you are very picky about what you eat and sometimes you just don't want anything. All you can do then is wait until you get a very clear signal to eat something you really want to eat, and you may be surprised at how little food it takes to satisfy you. This change may be very subtle, so keep paying attention. It's not a static change but may come and go so staying in tune is crucial.

## It's Up To You

One of the drawbacks of this recovery process is that all the decisions about what to eat and when to eat are left up you. You must think and act for yourself. Traditional diets typically take a lot of the guesswork out of dieting. In fact, one woman who'd just lost 18 pounds in six weeks on a diet in a magazine, (*way* too fast, by the way), commented that the diet was great for her because it left no room for error—she didn't have to *think* about anything—just do exactly what the diet told her to do. This may sound like a perfect plan to some but it is utterly unrealistic for lasting success. Can anyone live the rest of her life eating only and exactly what someone else allows her to eat while living in the food environment we have today? I don't think so.

The disadvantage of having all the say-so about your eating is that you have to take total responsibility for it—for the things that work for you and for the things that don't. This is hard for many people. It's easier to follow instructions and then, if things don't work out in the long run, blame yourself, which is usually the case, or blame the diet. There's no blame to go around here, unless you want to blame me. But I'm not going to tell you to apply these principles to your life and I'm not going to guarantee you'll succeed if you try it. It's up to you.

I'm often asked what I eat. I usually keep this information to myself because the question reflects the old diet thinking that there's a magic formula or food combination that will bring the desired results. What I eat has nothing to do with what you will learn to eat in order to normalize your relationship with food, with your body and your weight. Every body is different and every recovery is different. The principles for recovery are basically the same, but if you try to recover with rigid expectations, resistance to making necessary changes, and an unwillingness to keep your efforts aimed at managing *your part* of the recovery process, you will probably be disappointed.

There is one thing about my eating that I do share. I eat all kinds of foods that aren't typical for specific meals. I often have leftovers from the dinner the night before for breakfast or brunch. Then I might have eggs mid-afternoon and a big salad for dinner. I don't follow the rules here because I'm following my appetite.

## Illustration of Recovery:

Recovery begins with the end of the feast or famine cycle—the last feast. Remember, the cycle must end with a feast—the very last one you will experience. It may be a mild feast or a protracted one, depending on your recent diet history. Here's an illustration of what recovery looks like. Keep in mind that the stages may overlap and do not necessarily happen in order. This will give you a path to keep yourself going in the right direction in your recovery. If you get off track, you will know it soon enough by checking this simple illustration of the broad stages of recovery.

**Illustration of Recovery**

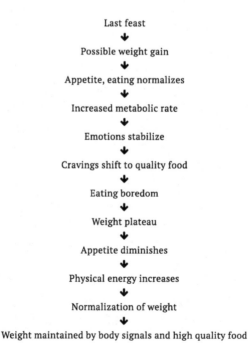

Last feast
↓
Possible weight gain
↓
Appetite, eating normalizes
↓
Increased metabolic rate
↓
Emotions stabilize
↓
Cravings shift to quality food
↓
Eating boredom
↓
Weight plateau
↓
Appetite diminishes
↓
Physical energy increases
↓
Normalization of weight
↓
Weight maintained by body signals and high quality food

## EXERCISE!

OK, here it is, what you've been waiting for—expecting all along: The key to recovery! You have to eat great food—yes, but you have to work out three hours a day—right? Wrong.

### Exercising for Weight Loss

We all need regular exercise and most of us need more than we've been getting. But there is a problem with our emphasis on exercise as a method of weight loss without any attention to eating enough good food.

We've established that famines—not eating in response to hunger signals—set people up to overeat later. When this is a regular pattern, it's called the feast or famine cycle. Now famines can be mild, moderate or severe, depending on two things: the degree of food deprivation and the level of physical activity. For dieters the degree of food deprivation depends on the diet. Often, dieters exercise along with eating less food. They do this to speed up the weight loss, but something else happens along the way. The combination of food deprivation plus high activity can create a *severe famine*. Without the exercise, this dieter might be in a mild or moderate famine, but the exercise makes the famine more severe and is even more likely to hook the body's survival response.

Does this mean that people should not exercise when they need to lose weight? *Absolutely not.* It simply means that people who exercise to normalize their weight must do it while eating a balanced quality diet.

Let's go back and look at the basics—the framework of adaptation. Fat accumulation is enabled by five biochemically-programmed adaptations: enhanced appetite, *lowered metabolic rate*, cravings, preoccupation with food and *avoidance of physical activity*. Inactivity helps promote fat accumulation and the need for excess fat promotes inactivity by lowering the metabolic rate.

If lowered metabolic rate and inactivity are important ingredients in the accumulation of excess fat in a person on the feast or famine cycle, then doesn't it make sense that increasing your metabolic rate by eating enough, and raising your physical activity level would promote fat loss? Back in diet land, you were trying to control your food intake and exercise more all at the same time, to burn calories. That probably led to pretty fast temporary weight loss. Now, we know you were shooting yourself in the foot, depressing your metabolic rate by not eating enough and actually promoting the very cycle that kept your fat going, at least in the long run.

These adaptation principles are a completely different approach because you are finally giving your body the nutrients and calories it needs *to be able to sustain a healthy exercise program.* You won't start a program and then stop it when you get too tired and too hungry to keep going. When you're hungry, exercise is painful and if it's painful sooner or later you're going to quit. *The key to lasting weight loss is not forcing your body into an energy deficit, which it cannot sustain. The key is giving it what it needs—and exercise is one of those things*—so it can finally, gradually lose the unhealthy fat it has been forced to accumulate in spite of your efforts—actually, because of your efforts.

It's important to know this because exercise has been over sold as a weight loss tool. Exercise is quite limited as far as weight loss goes. Bodies are designed to use fuel efficiently. Clinical research pioneer, Per Bjorntorp offered this example: The Vasa-loppet, a 49-mile ski race in Sweden that lasts approximately 10 hours, requires the energy equivalent of only two pounds of adipose tissue. Two pounds!

When I had foot surgery, and was unable to walk or work out, I wasn't concerned about gaining weight. Why? Because my body naturally adjusted to my decreased activity level, lowering my appetite, and I *lost weight* from not using my muscles. Go figure. Naturally, I regained the weight as I became more active.

Even with exercise, your body is a conservation machine, when you think about it. You can run on a treadmill for an hour and only burn a few hundred calories! Just compare that with the 10 minutes it takes to eat the small piece of chocolate fudge cake that contains 550 calories. No, bodies are built to conserve, and that's a good thing, really. Since you are not going to try to burn calories as a goal, just as you are not going to force your body to get along on a lot less food than you need, you are free to exercise for the health and the fun of it. You probably never thought about it that way, did you? Well, if exercise doesn't burn many calories, is it really so important for losing weight?

## Ladies and Gentlemen, Start Your Engines

We all know that exercise stimulates your metabolism, besides burning calories especially as you are active. But did you know that the stimulation of your metabolic rate does not stop when you stop exercising! Your engine is revved up and it stays in a higher than normal gear after you have left the gym or finished your walk. How much is it stimulated, and for how long? That depends on two things: how hard you worked out and how long you worked out. How hard you exercised is the most important variable here, and then the length of your exercise time is a factor too. Studies show that metabolic rate can remain elevated for several hours. The other thing to keep in mind regarding benefits of exercise is that muscle requires more energy to maintain than fat, so as you build up your muscles and use up your fat, your body will have to support those extra muscles with food. Muscular people can actually eat more food to maintain their weight than non-muscular people. This is another way your recovery will promote greater energy use overall.

Now, off the cycle and firmly in to recovery, you will want to exercise. Moving around more will finally feel good and right and do-able.

So, what kind of exercise are we talking about? The best exercise, according to experts today, is the kind that you will actually do consistently and is sprinkled throughout the day. Also, it's important that you enjoy it for the most part. This doesn't mean that spending time at the gym isn't really good. But, a mostly sedentary lifestyle plus formal workouts several times a week isn't as effective as doing spurts of activity throughout each day along with "formal" exercise. What are these "spurts" of exercise? You probably know some of them: parking away from a store entrance and walking the distance; taking the stairs whenever you can; doing jobs at home that require lifting or taking the stairs, i.e. carrying laundry baskets, turning commercial breaks into get up and move breaks; cleaning; lawn care; gardening; using work breaks for eating *and* moving around; parking a block or two from work. These changes in your everyday activity level will take commitment. It's just easier to park close, take the elevator, and sit through the boring commercials. You're probably used to that, but that doesn't mean you have to stay where you are. You can get used to something new, something much better, and it won't hurt because you won't be hungry.

Physiology expert, Dr. James Rippe, said, "Exercise haters need to change their mindset about what constitutes exercise. Exercise doesn't' have to mean going to a gym. Making a conscious effort to be more active all day can be more effective than running to the gym for twenty minutes and remaining sedentary the rest of the day."

## What About Cardio?

Recently, I asked a client about her activity level. She said she was walking the dog every day for about 40 minutes, but, she added, it wasn't "cardio." I supposed she meant that her heart rate wasn't being pumped up to a goal range and maintained there for a specific duration, so somehow it was inferior as far as exercise goes. Really? This mindset, that exercise must be strenuous sweat-producing and time-consuming to" count" has kept a lot of people from moving around more because they think it doesn't qualify as real exercise. Real exercise is body movement of any kind. You are exercising when you brush your teeth.

Workouts that are considered "cardio" stimulate the heart to beat harder and faster for cardiovascular conditioning. This is a worthwhile goal to do if you are healthy enough for it, and you don't need to exercise in this way for prolonged periods. Studies show that *twelve minutes* of aerobic exercise at an appropriate intensity, three tines a week, will offer you significant health benefits. It conditions your body to a heightened physical state and there are many benefits to cardio workouts. If you are unsure about your fitness level, check with your doctor before trying this more intense level of exercise. By all means, start exercising at your top potential and work up from that as you go along. When you expect more you usually do more and then you're likely to get more.

Our bodies are designed for much more movement than our American environment usually allows. Ideally, we need to be moving most of the day, so when we do get a chance to exercise in spurts, at the gym, or just walking in a park, we need to make the most of it. One thing we have to get over is this idea that activity doesn't count unless it is a certain type, reaches an intensity goal or fits somebody's description of "true exercise." My motto is "everything counts so start counting everything." Make it a challenge. How much extra movement can you fit into a day? Can you walk down the block? Can you put a CD on and dance while you're fixing supper? Can you walk the whole mall even though you only need to go to one store? Can you go up and down and up and down the stairs in your home or at your office? Lift weights during commercials? Remember, everything counts so count everything. Keep track of your physical activity every day if that helps keep you motivated.

## Habit

The dictionary defines habit as a custom, practice or routine. The example it gives is this: It was his habit to go for a run every morning. Breaking certain habits is difficult, but establishing them is hard, too. It takes decision, effort and conscious thought to turn a desirable behavior into a habit. First of all, you must consider the new behavior valuable to you, valuable enough to accept the inconvenience to you. You have to be convinced, at least on some level, that taking on a new habit is beneficial. If you have always thought of exercise in terms of losing weight, then this idea of activity spurts may seem insignificant, even ridiculous. But, research has spoken on this one and spurts of activity throughout the day—even for as brief as one minute—have benefits to overweight people and everyone, health-wise and weight-wise. Just get started and it could easily become habit-forming.

## Joining a Gym

If you want to join a gym, do it. Get a personal trainer, if you can. Gyms and trainers can be helpful, especially for getting you started on fitness goals and work out equipment. It's not necessary to do these things in order to succeed in recovery, but they can be helpful in keeping you committed. Talk with someone at the gym about your work out goals. It's best to avoid setting weight-loss goals because that will probably lead to a diet or some form of artificial control of your food intake. If the trainer is good, she will not expect quick weight loss, but *may* expect weight loss at a certain pace. The thing you seek at a gym is an environment of support in your commitment to improved conditioning, gradual weight loss and overall better health.

If you can't join a gym, don't worry about it. Get a treadmill or another all-body machine and a set of weights. Used equipment is available! No problem if you don't have any equipment. There are many great workout DVDs on floor routines that don't require anything but a floor. Buy or rent these and find the ones you like, that fit your body and needs. The best way to stay with your regular workout routine is to recruit a friend or relative to workout with you. Stick with a schedule— at least three or four days a week.

One practical way to make exercise fun is to associate it with something you enjoy. For example, I love stand up comedy, so I've set up my treadmill and weight set in front of my TV and watch comedy acts I've recorded while I work out. I'm walking and laughing and lifting and laughing and the time goes right by. I actually look forward to working out because this is when I watch these funny programs. Exercising with a friend accomplishes the same thing; if you're walking you're talking too. Dancing is fun and great exercise. You don't have to go to a club to do it—although that would be great too. Many of us have our favorite dance recordings and no one's stopping us from rocking out in the living room. Headphones are popular exercise equipment because they add fun music to any form of solo working out.

Just plain walking is good exercise, and for many people, the most convenient. Again, having a buddy is helpful to keep you on track. Walk in a mall if the weather is bad. Have a specific time on specific days to go. This applies to the gym, the DVD workouts, walking, running and whatever else you may do. Again, the best exercises are the ones you enjoy, and many people get moving doing a sport they like: golf, tennis, soccer, badminton, baseball, racket ball, and football. But, you have to *plan* it and then *do* it, and do it consistently!

Maybe you're out of shape and feel that almost any exercise is too much for you. Get a check-up with your doctor. Start slowly and build up your body and your time. It may not feel comfortable at first, but, like any good habit, it will get better as you get better. Start at five minutes, if that's where you are. Then, go to seven minutes, then 10, then 13, and then 20. This way, you won't experience so much resistance and are much more likely to keep going. Reaching small goals can be so reinforcing. If you can start at 15 minutes, or a half hour or even an hour, go for it, but make sure you can keep it going. Consistency is the issue here—and common sense.

Remember, besides the benefits that you and your body will enjoy from regular exercise, you are sending an important message to your body: Excess fat is now maladaptive, meaning it does not support survival. Consistently eating well and enough, and exercising more, tells your body to stop storing fat and then get rid of it. This doesn't happen in a hurry, but gradually your body will get the message.

Some of my clients are concerned that exercise increases their appetite, and wonder if they should eat more food to satisfy this change. This uncertainty stems from the old idea that eating more food automatically causes weight gain or prevents weight loss. Of course, if your appetite increases, you must satisfy it with a bit more good food. Otherwise, you may end up with symptoms of the feast or famine cycle. The cravings might start. Always keep up with your hunger by eating great food, but be on the lookout for that dip in your potions. You can trust your body to handle exercise too.

If you start an exercise plan and then you find yourself sloughing off, missing days and then weeks, change things up. Something isn't working and it's important to find out what it is. If you don't think about it, it will go away, and then you'll lose out on all the benefits. Talk it over with a friend. Explore your options. Don't just sit there—do something else!

## Eating Out

There's just no way to get around eating out. We all do it, for better or for worse. The better is obvious: The table is prepared by someone else. The food offered includes choices that never come out of our own kitchen. Everyone can choose whatever he/she wants. The food is delivered by a smiling person who treats you like you deserve all their attention. And, the table settings all belong to the restaurant so we can leave all the dirty dishes without any guilt whatsoever. We are not responsible for anything but the bill, and it's a bargain for what we get.

All that's the good part. But there are a couple of drawbacks. Many dieters confront their demons at a restaurant, and fall off their program. We know why. They are too hungry. They have been too "good" on their diets, keeping their eating limits carefully, downplaying their hunger.

You, however, are doing things differently now. You don't have to be intimidated by going out to a restaurant. It can be a pleasant experience, not a threat to your commitment to eating right, because of the sane and healthy way you've been eating all day long. But, you have to pay attention to some basic guidelines. First, let's talk about food quality at a restaurant, because it can be a problem. Quality is not the top priority in a restaurant. Taste is. And how can a restaurant enhance the taste factor? By adding fat in the form of butter, oil, sauces, cream, fatty meats, fried foods, and deep-frying foods—you get the picture. You've probably tasted the picture. Then, there's the salt and the sugar—okay already.

There will come a time when these fatty, rich foods will not appeal much to you anymore, but until that happens, what will you do? You will make sure to eat every time you get hungry throughout the day, including the few hours before you go. You will pay attention to the menu because you are not overly hungry, and you will order the best-quality food that you like from the menu. Maybe it won't be a perfect food choice, but it will be much better than you used to order and it will improve each time you go out.

For example, you like fried calamari for an appetizer, but you also like crostini or shrimp. This is easy. The grilled chicken salad sounds good but the half-pound California burger with cheese sounds really good, too. As long as you are not too hungry, this will be a manageable decision. You *know* the salad is much better food in terms of quality, but a salad doesn't really appeal to you. What else sounds good? A grilled chicken sandwich with cole slaw is your next best pick. Try each time to go with the best choices you can, shooting for real food choices—clean food.

Suppose you've gone to a movie with friends and they want to go out for pizza afterwards. Do you run home because you "can't eat after supper"? Do you go? Do you have an anxiety attack? No, your recovery should be sane and rational. Of course you go and, since you've eaten well all day long, you are not particularly hungry. This is why you didn't have the barrel of buttered popcorn and gigantic Coke at the movie. If you are hungry, have a piece of pizza, preferably the lighter variety, and enjoy yourself. If you find you aren't satisfied with that, then perhaps you haven't been paying close enough attention to your hunger during the day. Check it out.

## Discipline

This may sound like a dirty word to you when it comes to your eating. "Here we go—control yourself!" But that's not what I'm getting at.

My mother used to go out for lunch with her friends every Wednesday. One day, the topic of dieting came up and her friend, Millie, who was always struggling with her weight, asked her how she stayed so slim.

My mother said, "I don't know. I've always been thin."

Then Millie looked at her, almost accusingly, and said, "Peg, you're just disciplined, that's all. Look at your plate, you only ate half your sandwich! I wish I had your discipline."

What Millie didn't know was that my mother almost always ate something before she went out to eat because she didn't like to feel overly hungry when she ordered and waited for the food to arrive. By the time her food came, she could never eat the whole meal. She had spoiled her appetite.

I once did a seminar with chemical dependency coach Jeff VanVonderen. We had lunch with the other team leaders at a wonderful Italian restaurant. I ate almost half a plate of seafood fettuccine and Jeff remarked, "Aren't you going to finish that?" I told him I was full and he said, "So what? You are the only person I've ever seen voluntarily leave half a plate of seafood fettuccine on your plate—great seafood fettuccine!" But I just couldn't eat any more—I'd had an English muffin two hours before lunch.

## Portion Control

If your body satisfaction signals are the only guide to stop eating, does portion control factor into your recovery?

This program is based on biology and common sense. The trouble is that there is so much confusion and misinformation about food and eating that biology is ignored and common sense isn't so common anymore. So, the buzzwords "portion control" have made their way into this book.

Many people, including professionals in the obesity research field, blame the large portions in restaurants and bakeries for the obesity epidemic in our country. If this is true, then everyone who goes out to eat should be fat. But they're not. Many people just eat a part of the portion served them at a restaurant, and divide up the gigantic croissant from the bakery among two or three people. Why is this? Do they just have better willpower? And why do other people manage to eat the entire, overlarge servings and then have dessert, too? By now you should be able to answer these questions.

What to do about portion control? Satisfy your appetite with high quality food all day long every day. Never go to a restaurant overly hungry. If you are hungry before going to the restaurant, eat something light that will carry you through until the food actually appears on the table. Take something to drink or eat with you in case there is a delay while you are waiting to get in to the restaurant and you become very hungry. In this way, you accomplish some important goals. First, you will be able to order better-quality food. Second, you won't be tempted to eat the entire basket of bread with butter before the meal comes—in fact, you will be able to skip it so you can enjoy the great food you ordered. Third, when your food does come, you will savor it and enjoy it instead of desperately wolfing it down because you feel you are going to pass out if you don't. And fourth, you will be able to smile at the waitress who offers the dessert menu and say, "Thank you, I'm just too full."

This is where portion control comes from—all the eating that came before. The only time a person in recovery can consciously limit her/his food portions is when they get stuck after they are off the feast or famine cycle but they have not experienced a decrease in their appetite. In this situation, they need to back off on their portions and eat a bit less, gradually adjusting their diet to accommodate their bodies' need for less fuel.

## Getting Off Track

It is unrealistic for most people to experience a steady one-way recovery. The principles in this program are difficult to apply for many reasons. A serious one is diet propaganda. Those who recover have to completely block out the fast weight loss gimmicks and tricks on TV and magazines stacked in grocery store check out shelves, not to mention Internet diet ads. They must focus their goals and expectations on almost entirely different things. Recovery is holistic.

The focus of your recovery is you as a complete person, including your overall health and best weight. Many who have recovered say it's about getting your whole life back.

It only makes sense that people would struggle with ideas so contrary to everything they have believed for most of their lives. The idea that eating really good food, never going hungry, and letting your body tell you to stop eating, is bizarre to many, amazing to some, crazy to others. But if you see the sense in this approach and want to give it an honest try, keep reading! There are some wonderful things ahead.

# CHAPTER 9

## Losing Weight For Good

"Until one is committed there is hesitancy, the chance to draw back, always ineffectiveness. Concerning all acts of initiative there is one elementary truth...the moment one definitely commits oneself, then Providence moves too.

**—W. N. Murray of the Scottish Himalayan Expedition - 1951**

We've talked about food, we've talked about hunger, we've discussed exercise, we know about food availability and the feast or famine cycle and we've pretty much proved that dieting is bad for you. Now let's whittle it down to the core. Let's describe this program in a nutshell, contrasting it to the diet approach.

Traditional dieting approaches overeating and weight gain from theoretical causes such as emotions, stress, the availability of too much food, bad food, lack of discipline, laziness and gluttony. Although some of these variables may be relevant, the solution of this approach typically and oddly targets only the physical problem of excess weight. It proffers food-intake control plus exercise as the solution—forced weight loss based on the calories in/calories out theory. It requires unnatural will power and self-denial, which determined dieters employ in sometimes heroic efforts to lose weight fast. The big advantage of traditional dieting is the relatively rapid loss of weight, and this is why people keep doing it. The disadvantage is that weight lost by this method is almost always regained.

The adaptation paradigm demonstrates that overeating and weight gain are adaptive when food intake is intermittently limited. It is a holistic approach, targeting the underlying biological forces that lead to overeating and the accumulation of excess fat. Its principles are supported by research. There are many advantages to this approach: First, over weight people are not required to starve themselves in order to lose weight quickly. Hunger is satisfied, food choices are broad, patterns of recovery are established as guidelines, regular exercise is personalized and may be moderate. There are three basic drawbacks of this approach: It requires independence and strong personal commitment over time. It lacks structure; there is no diet to go on or off. The third drawback of this approach is that it takes more time to lose weight. The main advantages are lasting weight loss and freedom from the diet lifestyle.

**No Limits—Really?**

As I mentioned above, one of the distinguishing features of this approach is that there is no specific diet to follow; no one tells you when to eat, what to eat or how much to eat. This is usually more of a problem than not. Is this surprising? We've mentioned that dieters tend to want the structure of a legalistic program. There are so many decisions to make and dieters are not confident in their ability to make these decisions—just look at the sorry state their bodies are in when they decide for themselves! They want information on perfect foods, evil foods, vitamins, supplements, food combinations, fat burning foods, special recipes, and especially how fast they can lose weight if they follow the diet religiously. But besides their lack of confidence, I have noticed that dieters also have brains, experience, desire, learning potential and common sense. I believe those motivated to apply these principles will learn to shop, learn to eat, learn to relax about food and finally, learn to live in a new way. All along the way they will make this program their own because it is not a static one size fits all program. Each individual will work through the stages of recovery thoughtfully and patiently, the only way it can be done.

### If You Have Recently "Succeeded" on a Diet

The best time for people to embark on this program is when they are at their top weight and have been stable at that weight for a while. This is because their fat-stimulating biochemicals are not riled up from dieting—remember lipoprotein lipase? When these biochemicals are satisfied and their bodies have the fat they need, they are in a neutral zone, out from under the influence of famines and the fat production famines provoke. This is the situation for people who have completely rebounded from their most recent diets.

For dieters who have lost weight more recently and are thinking about applying these principles for the first time, this information is particularly relevant. The only way off the feast or famine cycle is on the feast side, so those who have most recently lost weight on a diet are biologically set up to gain that weight back. In other words they have to feast before they can end the war with their bodies. This is a little complicated so let's put it another way.

We understand that the famine experience in famine sensitive people always stimulates the production of biochemicals that cause fat storage. The main reason for excess fat storage is protection against starvation. Getting off the feast or famine fat producing cycle boils down to eliminating these fat-producing biochemicals so eating and activity can normalize. You know the only way to do this. Many people who start their recovery have recently been in some type of diet famine. So what happens when they start their recovery by eating according to their body signals? They may tend to overeat, and depending on their diet history and famine sensitivity, they may gain weight. What? Even on high-quality food? Yes.

If you have recently lost, say, 50 pounds on a diet, *your body is set up to regain that weight* in order to protect you from famines in the future. Your body doesn't "know" you're never going to famine again. It must prepare for the future based on your eating pattern in the past. Therefore, you may experience initial weight gain. If you are in this position, you may even gain all the weight back that you lost. Even great food will not prevent this rebound because *diet rebound is physiologically driven*. Some people who learn about the adaptation principles try to maintain their weight loss by continuing to diet, but they inevitably gain all the weight back and then start their recovery.

It's probably difficult to accept the possibility of weight gain at the beginning of recovery if you have recently lost weight dieting, but when you consider the near 100 percent likelihood that you will regain that weight anyway, it may be less painful. I am often asked the question: Can a person who has recently lost weight on a diet just apply the principles to maintain that weight loss? That may be possible, anything is possible. But the need for excess fat is so crucial for survival in environments where famines occur regularly, that bodies use any type of food to store fat. This means bodies can use food on the Real Food list. Studies have demonstrated that people do gain weight on a high quality food diet, and this is why they do. Our ancestors stored extra fat on their bodies in preparation for famine and they had only raw plant and animal foods with which to accomplish this. They had no pastries or fried chicken or ice cream or Nachos.

Does this mean you might as well eat food from the Borderline and Pleasure lists since you're going to gain weight anyway? I don't advise it for three reasons. First, it is essential to learn to choose only quality food from the very beginning because this is one of your top skills in recovery. Even if you gain at first, you are practicing making the best choices. Secondly, your nutritional status needs some attention if you've been dieting, and you will recover that the quickest on quality food only. Thirdly, you can minimize your weight gain and send your body the right message: Quality famines are over.

## Can You Speed It Up?

Just because weight loss is a good thing doesn't mean it is stress-free for bodies. Actually, there is a natural resistance both to weight loss, and weight gain because of this principle. Because of this natural, biological resistance to change, adaptive weight loss *must be gradual.* It is the abruptness, the fast-forced weight loss of traditional diets that violates this biological principle and sets dieters up for rebound. Bodies adapt slowly if the change is to last.

You will notice that the suggestions for speeding it up are basically the same for recovery in general. There are some adjustments anyone who is stuck can make to get their body moving toward weight loss. These speed-it-up techniques should be applied carefully, paying close attention to signs of the feast or famine cycle. If the cycle gets started as a result of trying to move things along faster, you may be pushing your body along too hard, so back off and go more slowly.

1.  Improve the quality of your food supply. Increase vegetables and fruits and whole grains. Learn to juice foods you love if you

are interested. Make sure you're getting enough high quality protein foods and complex carbohydrates. Stay in touch with your body. If you want a huge bunch of grapes, do it!

2. Drink water between meals and snacks. Often, hunger signals are thirst signals, too. Drink something when you first feel hungry. Sometimes, a drink satisfies hunger for a while which means you were probably thirsty. Research has shown that the vast majority of people do not drink enough water and water is a necessary element in burning fat.

3. Limit meals away from home to one or two a week. Your food quality may be taking a significant dip nearly every time you walk into a restaurant. Even if you order well and you're not too hungry, it's very hard to keep the food very high quality. Research the best places to get good food when you do go out.

4. Get 30 to 45 minutes of some type of exercise every day possible. Get 7 or 8 hours of sleep every day. Make these top priorities.

5. Attack old mindless habits. Used to finishing your food? Used to always taking the last bite? Used to two pieces of toast with your eggs? Get over it.

6. Fine-tune your unique body signals. Thirsty? Tired? Stiff neck? Need a stretch. Need a nap? Get to know all your body's signals intimately and take good care of it.

7. Back off on your portions. Once off the cycle, you are safe to consciously eat less food. You may find you need to eat more often, but maybe not. Take each situation as a separate experience. If you start to have cycle symptoms, ease up a little and try again in a week or two.

Does this look like a diet to you? It does to some people because of the suggestion to focus on some types of food, consciously eat less at times and exercise every day possible. Well, permanent weight loss is not magic. Bodies must be provoked into letting go of fat, one way or another. We know all about the diet way, forcing the fat off. But this way, enabling your body to use up fat because it doesn't need it any more takes just as much, perhaps more, effort. It certainly takes more time and that's why it doesn't backfire.

The part of recovery that will never even remotely resemble a diet is the prescription to eat all the high quality food you need to satisfy hunger as you break the feast or famine cycle. And only then, to carefully limit portions as your body tolerates it. Other programs suggest improving quality, but none suggest, much less require, that hunger be consistently satisfied, especially strictly at the beginning. This is the bedrock of this program. Without the consistent satisfaction of hunger to stop the war with your body, any program will lead back to the feast or famine cycle.

## Will I always have to be so careful to eat on time and only eat great food?

Probably, although perhaps not as strictly as while you are losing weight. At any rate, it won't feel so foreign to you after you've lived this way for a while. It will seem as natural as breathing. And besides, it's the best way to treat your body! Hunger causes stress—a kind of discomfort—that can be relieved. And the best and only reasonable way to relieve it is to eat! We have been trying to get around this for so long that it almost seems unnatural to us.

There will never be a good reason to go back to calorie counting or any other diet-type behavior. You may get off-track from time to time because of schedules, laziness or old under eating habits. You may get out of sync with your body, with your hunger and fullness signals, and you may get back on the feast or famine cycle. You may gain some weight but you'll know exactly what to do, and that *won't* be to go on a diet! You will go back to the basics and your body will get back to normal all over again, without excess hunger and without all the craziness of dieting.

## Relentless Interferences

Many people wonder if recovery is still possible if things like schedules continue to interfere with eating good food on time. Perhaps they can't stay off the feast or famine cycle because of these problems. When they get stuck and realize they are not practicing the basics of recovery, they are often surprised. They admit they eat late, they eat poor-quality food regularly, and they are not consistently active. It may be difficult to keep these things going in life, but recovery has to be a priority. The point is, you may improve your eating to a degree but if you are still sloppy in the other basic principles, you may never lose weight or keep it off.

Every individual must decide for herself how carefully she must adhere to this program in order to recover—to lose weight and enjoy a normal relationship with food. If after some months, there is no tolerance for lowered food intake, no change in appetite, cravings or energy level, then something is wrong. The "speeding it up" list is for you. Pay attention! There are situations in every person's life that interfere with applying these principles perfectly. These are unavoidable. So when you are able to control your eating and activity, they must come first. It's the *consistency of your effort* that will ensure your recovery.

## Still Thinking a Diet Might Be the Answer?

Many people experience "delayed enlightenment." It's interesting to me that quite a few people who read one of my books on recovery put it down, thinking, "That's interesting, but not for me, not now." Then, two or six or 10 years later, years of unsuccessful dieting, they pick it up and read it, and do it. Then, they contact me saying they wish they'd started sooner. Invariably, they didn't start sooner because they thought it would "take too long."

## When I Do Recommend Dieting

I am very careful never to push this recovery process on anyone who still feels as if dieting is the answer for them. I don't even encourage them to read the book. The reason for this is simple. People who still believe that there really is a diet out there that can lead to lasting weight loss must find it and do it. It's the speed of weight loss that is so alluring, as you know from your own experience, and it's a hard habit to break. So, I just bless those who are still headed in that direction.

## To Weigh or Not to Weigh, That is the Question

One challenging decision for people in recovery is whether or not to weigh them selves. Some choose not to weigh at all. This technique is helpful because it keeps the focus off the part that your body is supposed to do—burning the fat. If you don't know what you weigh, it may help you stay with your primary responsibility to satisfy your hunger with great food. It will protect you from discouragement or panic if the numbers aren't what you want or expect. Those numbers can be a distraction, possibly derailing you and tempting you to take drastic measures to speed things along, like trying to eat less and ignoring your hunger. It's probably a better gauge of your progress to watch how your clothes fit. Fat is bulky, remember, so it takes up more space. You might not be losing at all by the scale because of gaining dense muscle weight from more exercise, but you are losing fat at the same time. This shift will show up in the fit of your clothes.

Others opt for weighing once a month because they're so curious and want to track their progress. This is fine, as long as you can give your body the time it needs and let the numbers be what they are—numbers. Again, avoid letting the scale run your recovery and your life. If you can't do this, stay off the scale. The only adjustments you should make as a result of the numbers are to apply the program basics better.

Many ex-dieters are used to weighing every day or at least once a week. These options are probably going to cause problems. First of all, lasting fat loss does not happen overnight or even steadily from week to week. Real fat loss occurs over months and is irregular for the most part. For example, Juanita weighed herself every day and was stuck in a plateau for seven weeks. She grew restless, knowing those numbers hadn't budged downward. In fact, she went up two pounds during that time. Finally, after all that waiting, her weight suddenly dropped down five pounds. It really wasn't sudden at all. It just took her body time to make the shift. Of course, you can weigh as often as you like, but because your goal is of the long-distance, lasting type, *it's much more prudent to keep your eyes up on your eating and the ultimate goal* instead of down toward your feet.

There are ex-dieters who do decide to weigh themselves in spite of the potential pitfalls. They find the numbers on the scale motivating— reminders of what they are doing and why. They tend to tolerate the inevitable lulls in weight loss well, and keep in mind the necessity of taking time. It's easy to find out if you fit into this category or if you should back away from the scale during your recovery. If you want to weigh yourself, just try it and see how it affects you. You'll know whether the scale is a tool or a temptation for you.

## It Takes Time

What does this mean? You've heard the word "gradually" often in this book, so you're probably already thinking, "How much time?" I wish I had a simple answer, but remember, every body is different and every diet history is different. Remember the landmarks of recovery? One person had a change in appetite within five months and lost more than 35 pounds over the next two years. Maybe that doesn't sound like much compared to the last diet you tried, but six years after losing that weight, this happy individual has never regained a pound. In fact, she's lost more weight.

Where were you five years ago? Two years ago? Were you dieting? Were you thinner? Were you heavier? Five years seems like a long time, but looking back, it has a different perspective. Knowing what it took you to get to the weight you are now, wouldn't it be worth changing paths in spite of the slower recovery? Can you see yourself in a year or two, or five, eating like a sane human being, free to satisfy your hunger, out from under the pressures of cravings for lousy food? This is the picture to hold up because it will give you patience and motivate you to keep doing something new for a change—something that will bring many health advantages that last.

It's hard to work at something that takes months and years to accomplish when others are "doing it" in days and weeks. (Suddenly, they will be all around you, losing five pounds a week.) But time is the tradeoff here and there's no way around it. If you think of all the time you spent gaining weight and dieting and gaining it back, then it just makes sense that your body is going to require some serious time to reverse the process for good. How much serious time? Think in terms of weeks to get completely off the cycle and into a rhythm of eating on time. Then, give your body time to make the necessary biochemical changes that go with an optimal food supply and lead to weight loss.

This will probably take some months for your body to adjust. Once your expectations get realistic, you'll be able to relax and do your job—eating right and staying active. All these things will reassure your body that it is safe to use up extra fat. When you reach your ideal weight, there is no maintenance plan to go on. Just keep doing what you have been doing all along—why wouldn't you?

## Coming From the Other Side—Anorexia

### A mother's perspective

This mother was understandably terrified for her daughter. She found *Breaking Out of Food Jail* on the Internet and read it with her daughter. Her daughter recovered from this debilitating illness by applying the adaptation principles and her mother reports that she is now doing extremely well, eating freely, preferring organic healthy food, including desserts. She says her daughter has learned to read her hunger signals, and she eats until she is comfortably full. On this journey, she did have anxiety issues as she learned to trust the program. The early days were the most difficult, as her body learned to cope with food again. There were a few anxious months when she did gain, but she could also think much more logically and clearly, enabling her to understand that the weight gain was temporary. She knew her body also had to learn to trust her again, and once it did, then her weight leveled off and has remained steady ever since—for four years.

I recently saw two photos of this young woman—one before and one after her recovery. The before picture is frightening. Now she is radiant and has a beautiful, natural figure.

Anorexia is considered to be a chronic, incurable illness.

**Debbie**

I became anorexic beginning at age 15 and continued off and on until I completely stopped starving myself at age 28. I went through some serious binging and starving, losing control of my eating, and not understanding why and what was happening with my body. Finally, I went to see a famous doctor who gave me the tools to help me get my body healthy again. But I was scared as I was going through the weight gain and the tight fitting clothes, and eventually I had to throw away the scale because I didn't want to see what my weight was anymore.

It wasn't until I came across your wonderful books, that I was *completely* convinced about how a body works and why it goes through what it goes through when it's starving. Your book totally hit the nail on the head. Now mind you, I'm not taking anything away from the doctor who helped me. He did help me tremendously, but your book explained in detail the why's, the what's, and the how's which is exactly what I needed most. I needed to know why this was happening, and how I can prevent it from happening again, and what caused it to happen in the first place. I can't tell you how many "aha moments" I had when I read your books.

Thank you so very much for writing these wonderful books. I'm so happy that you did. If there was one person that you helped more than you know, it was definitely me.

**Becoming Who You Really Are**

In the process of recovery, you and your body merge into one identity. The person you knew was inside you will actually come out into the open, even before you lose all the weight you want. As you become secure in the process of your recovery, and completely free of the diet lifestyle, you will experience a tremendous freedom in your relationship with your body and with food. Naturally, the interval between enlightenment and new identity varies quite a bit. The range I've witnessed goes from a few months to one year for the mental/ emotional stability and one year to seven years to reach an ideal weight.

These time tables depend upon an individual's ability to stay off the feast or famine cycle and stay with high quality food.

Recovery is likely to be interrupted by life events that influence eating and appetite. Things that interfere with hunger, such as high stress and illness, may put an individual back on the feast or famine cycle. This can't be prevented sometimes, but these problems are self-limiting, so usually people pick up where they left off. For the recovering person, emotional difficulties may also interfere with eating and cause cycling. These problems may cause temporary weight gain, and although disappointing for the person in recovery, resolve themselves as life events settle down.

I have heard from a few people who have gotten off the feast or famine cycle, changed their eating behavior and food availability, and reached their ideal weight within months after starting. Naturally, these individuals are near their ideal weight when they start—usually not more than 10 pounds overweight. However, these relatively thin people often report that they had a history of disturbed eating patterns and were able to recover the freedom to eat normally.

## Claudia

I thought you might be interested to know how one of your readers made out by following your suggestions, which I wish could be put in the hands of every overweight person in America. I immediately began following your instructions and, at the same time, resurrected my somewhat lagging aerobics classes. Although I have never been obese, I have certainly had my share of issues around food, including cravings, and occasional bulimia. From the day I started your program, 18 years ago, I never had another problem—not one! I love good food and I eat a lot, particularly vegetables, fruits, whole grains, beans, and fish. I have almost entirely lost my cravings for sweets, they just don't interest me. I am never hungry, have loads of energy, and lost weight the first month, without looking at the scale, or even thinking about it. I lost 22 pounds during the first two years and I've stayed slim and bulimia free ever since."

Joanna's story may seem trivial to you if you have 40 or 110 pounds to lose. But it is relevant because the eating behavior, cravings and bingeing that plagued Joanna are the same ones haunting dieters everywhere. The food palate Joanna settled on is right in line with the recommendations here. And like others in recovery, she admits, "I love good food and *I eat a lot.*"

## About Evening Hunger

We've discussed the shift from eating most food later in the day to eating most food earlier in the day. People in recovery experience this shift, or at least should experience it, early on. Bodies naturally require most fuel intake during the hours of greatest activity, tapering off to less and less as activity wanes. Although this is normal and makes biological sense, it also makes sense that dieters tend to eat more at night and less during the day. Besides the feast or famine cycle influence, they need the fat that nighttime eating provides. Reversing this pattern is tantamount to recovery and requires diligence during the first months until it is well established. The last meal of the day, sometimes eaten as early as 4 p.m., according to some who have recovered, should be the last time of significant hunger.

## Connie

My first glimmer of hope came about seven weeks into my new routine. I was out to dinner and half way through my meal, I suddenly couldn't eat anymore of the delicious meal before me. I was so surprised that at first I thought I was getting sick. But then, when I realized I really didn't want any more, I burst into tears, right there in the restaurant. I think the waiter thought someone had died. I just couldn't contain the relief I felt—that my body could control my eating and actually stop me from eating more. The whole key for me was eating enough throughout the day, every day—something I never would have figured out in a million years! I still weigh less than I did most of the time [I was dieting], and now I can live and eat like a normal human being—I'm free!

Just what is "significant hunger at night?" It is hunger that calls for eating a substantial amount of food—more than just a light snack—to get comfortable. It is the hunger that tends to trigger make-up eating at night. And this type of hunger *should be a thing of the past if you are on track*. Remember, eating good food on time is the only way to prevent excess hunger and the overeating that goes with it. This is the whole focus of recovery: eating good food on time so that you can make good food choices consistently, avoid nighttime and anytime overeating and lose weight.

Strong hunger at night is usually a symptom. Either you've not kept up with your hunger during the day, you are not completely off the feast or famine cycle, you still have rebound weight to gain back from a diet in the recent past, or you have been more active than usual. Always look at nighttime hunger as a symptom and try to diagnose it so you can fix the problem. It is possible, at least early on, that the hunger you experience in the evening may have to do with the long-standing physical response of your body to having food at that time. Your stomach may actually anticipate digestion in the evening if this has been a common time for you to eat. In this case, a retraining may be necessary to hurry your body along to exclusive daytime eating. To retrain your body, it's best to avoid eating at night right from the start, and to be consistent in this. The sooner your body gets used to the healthy emptiness of the period following the last meal of the day, the better.

What about light hunger? Light hunger at night is easily managed by some light food such as fruit, a few nuts or, yogurt. It's better to ignore light hunger at night, if you can still sleep.

## Other Patterns of Eating

Is the five-meals-a-day pattern necessary? The "six small meals" approach has been around for quite a while. What if I don't fit into this pattern?

There is no set script for people in recovery. The five meals notion comes from the feedback I get from most of the people I've counseled over the years who have recovered. It applies to me. But it is only necessary for you to plug into the basics and you will find out what works for you. Some people who've started out on the three-meal-a-day plan find out that they really are hungry between meals—something they never really knew because they weren't looking for it. So, don't worry about other people's patterns—find your own.

## Complaints

What are the common difficulties and stumbling blocks to this approach? To some, at least at the beginning, it seems too good to be true—eat whenever you want, as much as you want until you're full. Of course, it's a little more complicated than that, as you know by now.

Oddly, in light of what I just said, the number one list of complaints of people starting out in recovery is: I have to eat all the time! It's boring. I'm constantly thinking about taking food with me. My hunger is relentless—I have to eat every hour and a half! It's interfering with my life. It's worse than dieting!

Many of these complainers have legitimate grievances but they recover just the same. The initial changes are particularly challenging. The struggle with change has to be countered by equally formidable traits.

After the effort of keeping an optimal food supply in place, waiting to lose and the uncertainty of whether or not you are "doing it right" are real difficulties for many. Probably the most challenging aspect of recovery is the patience required for weight loss. Also, the independence of recovery—that there are no weigh-ins or objective weight goals—makes it lonely for some.

Probably the most interesting complaint I've heard is this: Now that I'm eating well all day long, when I go out to dinner, it isn't special anymore. I'm not that hungry and I'm not particularly interested in ordering food I used to love to eat. It's a little disappointing to tell you the truth. It's just another meal, and I don't even want dessert. I take half the food home but usually end up throwing it out. I kind of miss the old dinners out.

## Does This Program Work for Everybody?

No.

The adaptation principles can be applied by anyone, but this program is not for everyone. Although the approach is simple on the surface, applying the principles to individual lives with all their unique circumstances is often complicated.

The two reasons people who understand, but consciously choose not to use this program are these: *it takes too long, and it's too much work.* We live in a culture of instant gratification and the diet industry is fraught with gimmicks offering quick, pain-free success. Even after many failed attempts, many dieters hold onto hope that there is an easier, softer way.

Some who try are unable to consistently apply the guidelines because it requires persistent effort, especially at the beginning when food choices and hunger satisfaction must become new habits. This sometimes proves to be too much for them. Others do not have consistent access to high-quality food, although they do benefit from learning to eat better food on time. And some, because of medical conditions, medications, or other reasons, are unable to lose significant weight. But, it is also possible that some bodies simply take more time to adapt, and as long as individuals keep working on the basics, they can succeed. Consequently, I never give up on anyone.

Some individuals simply cannot arrange their environmental food supply to stay satisfied with good food. Some have difficulty identifying their hunger and fullness signals. Very obese people tend to struggle with eating enough—and good enough—food consistently. Denial continues to play a role for many regarding food quality and the need for increased activity. Perhaps there are people whose bodies have gone through a permanent adaptive change so that their bodies are in a continuous state of readiness for famine. This would make lasting weight loss by this or any means unlikely. And, some people are addicted to dieting, to controlled under eating. They can't give up the controls long enough to enable their bodies to make the shift to readapting.

Although emotional eating is a misnomer, there is one emotion, which definitely affects eating behavior, and it is fear: fear of food, fear of weight gain, fear of losing control, fear of the unknown. For many, fear is the obstacle to overcome if they are going to leave the diet lifestyle for good and learn to eat in a sane and healthy way.

I have noticed that the ones who recover their normal relationship with food and normal body weight have some characteristics in common:

1. Clear understanding of the basic principles of adaptation
2. Confidence that dieting will never work for them
3. Perseverance—hold long-term goals over time
4. Independence—own their recovery
5. Common sense—able to troubleshoot and adjust
6. Discipline—keep choices consistent with recovery principles

Consistently applying these principles requires maintaining the paradigm shift away from the diet mentality. Those who recover must embrace a new mindset and cling to this change in their thinking as their recovery is established.

Are these principles so complicated that it takes a whole book for people to know what to do to recover? Not necessarily. I have counseled many clients in the basic principles without any book to support them in their journey. I did some coaching, but no more than an hour or two. These individuals applied the basics and experienced recovery on every level. They consider themselves naturally thin—they are naturally thin! Their maintenance program is the same as naturally thin people, essentially the same as recovery, although the quality food range may be broader. So, although recovery is complicated in some ways, it really boils down to some simple do-able ideas.

## Recovery Interrupted

Patricia recovered from decades of dieting after she met me at a party and challenged my ideas. There was no book to give her so I *told her* about the basics of adaptation and she could see that she had been on the feast or famine cycle for many years. So, she went home and started eating. Months into recovery Patricia started to go down in pants sizes. Her weight loss was temporarily delayed by a stressful family situation. During this difficult time—several years—Patricia was just focused on surviving. Her eating definitely took a back seat. But she did well anyway, stayed on a plateau for several years and then gradually continued to lose. Fifty-five pounds later and still diet-free, she knows there is no other way. Patricia went from a size 16 to an 8 and that was 25 years ago.

## Jasmine

Patricia and Jasmine's lives crossed when they worked in the same office for two years. Jasmine was obviously quite overweight and talked about every diet she tried. Patricia had to bite her tongue. Those who recover know better than to offer suggestions to dieters at any stage of dieting, unless they ask. Predictably, Jasmine lost weight and gained it back, lost it and gained it back again. It was hard for Patricia to witness this because she knew the struggle and frustration of chronic, unsuccessful dieting.

The last day Jasmine worked with Patricia, she said something surprising. She looked at Patricia and said, "You're really thin. You're always thin and you seem to always be eating. What do you do to stay so thin?" Patricia simply gave her the basics: Eat whenever you get hungry. Stop when you get full. Get some exercise every day. And give it time.

Two years later, a woman showed up in Patricia's office. She looked familiar but Patricia couldn't place her. "Do you remember me?" Jasmine asked. Patricia replied, "I think so, but I don't remember your name."

They had a good talk. Jasmine had lost almost 50 pounds over that time. Twenty-five pounds a year—two pounds *a month*! And yet, after two years, she looked like a different person. She thanked Patricia for her advice and told her it had not been that hard for her once she got over the shock of all that food. She didn't have to fear food or eating anymore. She just had to stay with the basics. *All she had to go on for her recovery were the basics.* No book, no training, no coaching, no nutritionist. Jasmine listened. She saw herself on the cycle. She got it. She did it. That was eight diet-free years ago.

## Where Do You See Yourself?

Jasmine was clearly ready for the information Patricia shared with her. *She had dieted herself to a point of open mindedness.* She had lost her hope, burned her bridges, and surrendered her delusions about dieting. *She knew* another diet was never going to help her for long.

Such absolute conviction is helpful but not required to recover. I've witnessed people who still entertained the possibility that some diet out there might bring the results they desired. But, they weren't sure, and they were open to trying something different, at least for a while. Many of these people got hooked on eating, leaving the pain of going hungry and the war with their bodies behind. And they saw changes in their eating and in their attitude towards food almost immediately. These experiences kept them hopeful and encouraged them to continue to apply these practical principles.

Where are you on this spectrum? The honesty with which you face your past experience with eat-less/exercise-more dieting will make the difference in your openness to this brand new way of thinking and eating. Are you open? Do you have even a little hope that there is something better for your body, for you, for your life?

There is.

# CHANGED LIVES

**(All names and some details here have been altered to insure privacy.)**

Having lived in the hell of eating disorders including bulimia, bingeing, and relentless dieting, I finally found a way out! My life was completely out of control before I learned about the feast and famine cycle and how it kept all that pain going. Now I don't know how I ever lived that way.

Nora

---

Getting free from the constant preoccupation with food was like a miracle to me. Even before I began to lose weight, I was so relieved! The freedom to eat like a normal person, to get hungry and then eat, period—I never thought it was possible for me.

Kelsey

---

This program wasn't like the diet clinics I'd been to before, that's for sure. And it was the total difference in Jean's approach that got my attention. The first surprise was learning to get in touch with my body. That was a huge change. Then I needed to learn to take the time to lose weight, but I was so convinced that that was no problem. I had tried so many weight loss programs over nearly twenty years and I knew another diet wouldn't work. It was a huge relief to find out that my crazy eating was biological and not emotional.

Veda

---

Over the years I had actually become afraid of food. This fear covered just about all food, but particularly fatty food and sweets. I was very careful about what I ate no matter where my diet was at the time— losing, gaining, or in a plateau. Now that I've lost the weight for good, I have a much more relaxed attitude about food. It doesn't scare me anymore. And when I have a dessert or sweet snack, I think, Big deal. I'd rather have a bunch of grapes!

Genette

---

Our culture is big on instant gratification. We want results now and that explains the thriving diet industry. We have a pretty warped idea of time and think we can lose weight in six months that took us 20 years to gain. Like Jean says, taking time to lose weight is the only sure way to keep it off, and that time spent adds up to long term sanity, besides a stable weight. Take the time now to get to a healthy weight. Once you get there, all you have to do to maintain it is to keep good food around and eat a wide variety. Without the strain of dieting, you'll be able to invest your energy into other more important things because you made the commitment to deal with you your eating/weight issue long before.

Peggy

---

I've been bulimic for over 12 years. I've been to treatment four times, and I've also been to therapy for over two years. I haven't really learned much from all this attention and support, but I've spent thousands of dollars over the years, not counting the insurance company contribution. I have had no relief from this plague, in spite of all this counseling.

I found out about the Naturally Thin recovery principles just a few weeks ago and, although I was skeptical, I tried the basic first step, to try to eat a little more when I got hungry. It became easier to eat more food more often and I was able to keep satisfying my hunger every time by week two. I had one last binge/purge episode at that time. That was it. That was the very last time I had a binged or purged. The last time, the very last time. I'm wondering, what was all that eating disorder treatment about?

Victoria

---

Nothing can keep me from my goal, so I've kept my weight and eating under control by sheer determination. I was one of those 'arrogant thins' that Jean talks about because I just gutted it out, starving myself to keep my weight under control. This kept me from bingeing even when I was dizzy with hunger. I played mind tricks on myself to keep myself convinced that I was eating enough when really I wasn't. It's crazy, in a way, but I convinced myself that I was on the right track, and it was the only way to keep my eating and weight under control.

Earning the right to eat was a big part of my program. In other words, I believed that I needed too burn a certain number of calories before I deserved to eat anything. So, before I learned how to eat like a rational person, I'd work out so I could eat. After I learned about this program, I eat to exercise. Fueling my body has become a priority and I eat frequently now, even every couple of hours. And I eat a lot, sometimes as much as 3,000 calories a day. Now my body and I are cooperating and it's a lot more fun! I've learned that if I don't do my part, my body can't do well. I eat a lot of great food. It's amazing the amount of food you can burn when you're naturally thin.

Roy

---

Certain foods have been off limits to me for a very long time. The cravings for these foods when I was dieting were almost overpowering. Now that I'm eating real food when I get hungry, if I want these 'pleasure foods,' only want them once in a while, where before the urge was every day. And the urge doesn't last like it used to. One cookie or a handful of chips and that's it! There's some kind of built in limit. My body just says 'no.' I can actually ask myself, is this really what you want? How is it going to make you feel? I can actually think these things through!

The changes have been gradual for me. I'm eating better, sticking with real food and making progress. Just a while ago I was eating a whole bag of cookies and half bag of chips.

Lauren

---

When I was on the Feast or Famine Cycle, my thoughts centered on food and my body almost all the time—nearly all my energy went into that. My main concern now is making sure I get enough good food, period. My weight is just right and stable. I feel a tremendous freedom that I never felt all those years of dieting and bingeing.

Kim

---

Jean, thank you for helping me understand my eating disorder and also accept the fact that I couldn't help doing what I did to try to stay thin. I have let go of the guilt that I have experienced over the years because it was simply ignorance that drove me to do the things I did. My self-rejection has been just as hard to bear as my disturbed eating but I have finally changed that. I am finally truly confidant that my life will be good. I wish you could see my heart right now. I feel it shines so much brighter because of the message you've brought. Thank you so much.

Janice

---

I was pregnant when I first read Naturally Thin. I had a long diet history so it really impressed me immediately. What a revelation! Your book changed my life and made it possible for me to lose 35 pounds over three years—all without dieting one day! I don't always follow the real foods, but I do eat on time and it keeps working for me!

Thank you—you have changed my life! I'm really happy, never depressed and the best thing of all—no more emotional eating!

Anna

---

When I started [my recovery] I was addicted to chocolate. I could not get through a day without a serious quantity. When Jean said I would lose my cravings for sweets when I learned to eat enough good food, I did not believe her. Maybe this could happen to other people, but not me.

Ten days into following the principles, I noticed that I had not had chocolate for three days in a row. I actually forgot about it. I knew then that my body could change too, if I learned to take care of my hunger. I was hooked.

Louise

---

I want the years I spent dieting back. We are so fortunate to understand this great program. There's nothing else like it anywhere! We have the key to eating in a normal, natural way. We will never have to diet or go hungry or starve or binge or obsess. Those days are over forever. I've just completed 7 years in recovery and I've lost all the weight I need to, mainly before my 4$^{th}$ year. Although my weight loss is pretty dramatic, most people are not open to the principles. I find that pretty amazing.

Winnie

---

I have been so out of control of my eating for so long that once I started this program I just assumed that I'd have the same problem. But then, somewhere during my sixth month when I was sure I'd eat and eat—and then I didn't. I couldn't! I was full. And it was just that simple. Oh my God.

I'm about two years in recovery and I am experiencing diet boredom. Don't know what I want, don't want anything, don't really want to eat at all. No cravings! I never get over the profound impact of simply eating enough good food when you need it. I am shocked that this is actually happening to me.

There is one truly amazing change I am going through now. I have always had a dread of food and eating, at least since I became a hard-core dieter. But since this diet boredom started, my fear and anxiety about food, which have plagued me for years, have pretty much disappeared. It's like eating is just eating. I never imagined I would feel like this. I can't remember a time when I ever have.

Sarah

---

Let me share how your work has impacted my life. I read your first book several years ago, and it gave me the foundation to recover from years of bingeing, dieting, self-starvation, eating disorders and tremendous guilt. I have been in recovery for 12 years—12 years of freedom. I am pursuing a career in nutrition counseling now and I'm excited about the opportunity to help others break free as well! I will happily be giving you and your work credit along the way. So thank you Jean!

Pauline

---

I had the opportunity to read your first book "How To Become Naturally Thin" in 2007 and I began in earnest to apply what I had read. "I am in the medical field and when I read your book it resonated with my professional education and my life long struggle with weight issues.

Having many different sizes of clothes has been a part of my life since I can remember. I am happy to say that after following the principles in your book for about 4 years I've finally at a stable and healthy weight. Thank you for settling the size I should be.

Roger

---

Thank you so much, Jean. Your book honestly saved my life! I was just starting medical school when I found it. I have been following your recommendations for the past 8 years. I am 31 years old; I have 2 boys, ages 3 and 5. Everyone in my family is overweight and they all think it's an accident that I'm thin. I brought your book home and read it cover to cover and immediately started practicing. It did take some time, but eventually I figured it out. I lost the weight and got my whole life back. Thank you so much!

Mia

---

My diet history began with a big diet organization and included diet pills (amphetamines), diet support groups, and a spiritual approach to dieting, to name a few. I began your program in 1995, when I was 47 years old. My last binge happened a week after I started. I was surprised that my appetite and relationship with food became normal within just a few months. I actually felt 'naturally thin' once my appetite normalized, even before I'd lost much weight. I dropped sizes slowly and erratically, leveling off during several crises in my life. I finally weighed myself at a size 10 and had lost 40 pounds, down from a snug size 16 to a 10 and then an 8. I was once miserably and hopelessly diet addicted, and now I really am naturally thin. You have to get right with food first, and the weight trouble gradually takes care of itself. You just can't believe it until it happens to you and then it's like waking up from a nightmare.

Lenore

---

I can personally attest that this recovery program has given me my life back. Life still gives me lemons from time to time, but my eating problems are resolved. What a difference it has made on my outlook on life!

Patty

---

When I first read about these principles, a light bulb literally went on in my mind and I made an instant paradigm shift in my thinking. I abruptly stopped counting calories. I realized how very important these ideas were, not just to me, but to everyone. I understood what was going on with my body and I had belief and hope that I would recover over time. And I did.

I was 51 years old when I found Jean Antonello's program and she truly saved my life. I was in denial about my eating disorder, exercising 24 hours some weeks, continually binging and gaining weight from it. I was so discouraged, many times thinking there was no hope. After I read her first book, I was so happy and I've never once had another binge. My weight has been stable, and I'm a size 6. I walk a lot and have plenty of energy to do it!

This is important information! Every dieter and even non-dieters need to know about how the body works. If we reach to even one person, who knows how big a difference we can make. I know. I'm living proof.

Melanie

---

I had been coping with food issues for almost fifteen years. I was on the feast/famine cycle all that time, but of course I couldn't figure out what my problem was. I thought I was just a really bad dieter. I couldn't understand why I didn't have the self-control to keep dieting and nothing explained why I went totally out of control at times.

Finally, the "food jail" I was in drove me to the end of myself. I just couldn't take it anymore—the relentless hunger and cravings and hating myself. And then one night in my despair, I found your book on the Internet. The moment I starting reading passages from your book, I began to understand everything. I cannot explain the relief that spilled over me. I got your book and read it cover to cover. I followed everything your said to do, as best as I could, not because I believed it would work, but because I just couldn't take it anymore and felt like I had nothing left to lose. I knew diets didn't work. And even though I was scared to let go and start eating again, and stop weighing myself, I just went with it because I knew my old patterns weren't working.

Everything happened just like you said it would. It took time—it wasn't a quick fix like a fad diet or a juice fast. Slowly but surely, I changed my whole lifestyle around eating over a period of months and years. I was able to change the way I ate—when I ate, what I ate, how much I ate—as well as how I thought about food, media, dieting, and body image. You said my "full switch" would turn back on, and it did. And I didn't think about food all the time, I didn't have to rely on a scale, and I eventually began to desire "quality" foods. The junk food cravings became less intense, portion "control" became natural and organic, and my body started to just plain work better.

Now, for the first time in a very long time, I honestly feel good about the way I look and feel. I don't feel hungry or deprived. I feel freed from food jail. It is an amazing sensation to realize I can eat whenever I am hungry, until I am satisfied—to be confident that I will know when to stop and happily certain that I won't gain weight. It's like I have inherited this huge estate with limitless assets.

Eventually my body took my weight to a place I never thought I'd be without strict dieting. I am thin. I am thin. I can eat. I can buy clothes without anxiety. I like how I look. I can eat. I can eat. I can eat. It's like waking up in an entirely new country—a country with loads of food and no restrictions.

I am so grateful. Jean, I have recovered from life-long food and eating problems—problems that made my life a living hell. Your program is simple in a way, but very frightening too. I had to let go of so many fears and prejudices to get better. I still struggle with some of the old nagging fears, but every day it gets easier, and every day I cherish the fact that I can live without food-guilt; that I don't have to diet; that I can feed my body. Thank you for helping me to change my life for the better.

Anastasia

---

I am one of those whose life was changed by your advice. It has been 10 years now since I lost weight on your program, starting at a size 12 and ending at a size 6. I am a size 6 every morning when I wake up and every evening when I go to sleep, and I am ever grateful to you for that simple but elegant fact. I still have no idea how much I weigh, which after all those years of obsessive attention just delights me. Your program has helped me in other ways, too, teaching me to trust my instincts and listen to my body on everything from sleep needs to career decisions.

Marjorie

---

I bought your first book on recovery by the principles of adaptation, *How to Become Naturally Thin by Eating More,* over nine years ago. I don't know why. I was a hard-core dieter, so I also bought another popular diet book. Your book didn't appeal to me at first because I wanted to *know* exactly what to eat and how much and I wanted to lose a certain amount of weight for a wedding I was going to be in. Well, I lost the weight on that diet, about 35 pounds in four months, and by the time a year rolled around, I was bigger than when I started. I remembered the feast or famine cycle from your book and figured I'd better take a look again.

That was eight years ago. I was at my all-time top weight. As I read your book, I became confident that I needed to stop dieting and learn to eat. At first, it was a struggle, choosing the best food and getting some exercise in most days. But about four or five months into it, I noticed my appetite changing once in a while—downward. Long story short, I learned to eat on time, to eat good food. I never binge, I don't worry about my eating or my weight, and I'm almost back to my weight as a high school senior, 132, (down from 165), before I started to diet. I've had to give almost all my clothes away, happily. I never thought I could really be naturally thin, but I am, and I have been *diet free* and thin for over six years.

Geneen

---

"I was an emotional overeater for years, gaining weight in spite of strenuous dieting. When I learned about [your program], it made sense to me instantly. My whole life was geared to staying away from food, and when pain or stress came along, my willpower broke down under the load. I finally saw why I binged when I got upset. I needed to binge. I was starving.

Learning to eat wasn't that easy for me. I was obsessed with dieting. But it was worth the effort. After two months, nothing made me want to binge anymore, and I had plenty of stress with three little boys. Even when my husband said he was leaving me for another woman, I tried to binge. But I couldn't do it. I couldn't overeat, so I just sat and cried and then I called my friend.

When problems came up after that, I just felt anxious, or sad, or mad, or worried. But I couldn't binge. Gradually, I lost the extra weight I'd gained by starving myself—a bonus I wasn't even counting on.

The thing that people need to understand about this program is this: When you get your eating straightened out, and stop starving yourself, much more than your diet is going to change. Your whole life changes in a way. I mean it. My entire life has changed because I finally learned to eat. I'm quite a different person. Ask anybody who knew me then and knows me now. I've changed."

Zoe

# APPENDIX

## The 31-Day Quick Start Plan

You have made a complete paradigm shift in order to understand and succeed on this program. As you know, this isn't a set of rules to follow; limits on food or food categories or required exercise regimens. It's a major shift in thinking—about your body, about food, about biological dynamics that cause cravings, overeating and metabolism problems. All this information has become a normal part of your thinking about your body.

But even if you're confident about the Naturally Thin® principles, you'll need some support for at least the first few months. I've written a blueprint here covering all the basics for you. Many in recovery have said reviewing the books has also been helpful to keep them on track and eventually over the finish line. Please read through the entire 31-day Quick Start first. Then take your reading one day at a time to focus on each individual principle.

You can do this. Stick to the basics. Don't get distracted by some new fad out there. And work hard—nothing as great as freedom comes easily.

DAY ONE
Key Theme: FREEDOM
OWNING MY DIET

I am responsible for my own body. I make the decisions that affect my body for good or bad. I enjoy the benefits and suffer the consequences of choices I make that affect my body. I am the only one who can make the choices that will ultimately result in my body's permanent and natural slimness. I am the only one who knows my body's hunger and other need signals. I am in control of the availability of food in my environment. I choose when, where, what, and how much I eat. Now I understand that these choices can lead to my becoming a normal, thin person. I choose to choose wisely.

"Self-trust is the first secret of success."

Ralph Waldo Emerson

Food for Thought: I have permission to eat well, every single day.

DAY TWO
Key Theme: FAITH
BELIEVING IN MY BODY

My body is the product of thousands of generations of human beings whose survival has been ensured through adapting to various levels of food availability. It is the accumulation of excess fat that has guaranteed human survival. My body has been working to keep me alive too, but now my body knows how to become slim. It has a built-in need to use up fat when it becomes unnecessary for its survival. I can make that fat unnecessary by eating exceptionally well every day. My body will do the rest.

"Reactivate the dynamic quality of confidence based on the realistic fact that you have the knowledge and the ability to do what needs doing . . .You know how to do it competently."

Norman Vincent Peale

Food for Thought: Getting slim *is* natural.

DAY THREE
Key Theme: HOPE
TAKING MY TIME

Think back to a year ago, two years perhaps. Does it really seem that long ago now? If you have been suffering from the Feast or Famine Cycle, you may think, *yes, it has been a long year.* Waiting to lose weight or gaining it back has a way of dragging on and on and on, especially when it's uncomfortable, even painful. But one or two years *without the pain* is not too big a price to pay to be cured of a lifetime of obesity. It is the best bargain around.

"We need some imaginative stimulus, some not impossible ideal such as may shape vague hope, and transform it into effective desire, to carry us year after year through the routine work which is so large a part of life."

Walter Pater

Food for Thought: Same time next year.

DAY FOUR
Key Theme: SKILL
FOOD AVAILABILITY CHECK

Check your Food Availability Factor for home, workplace, leisure, transportation, and travel/vacation. Examine the foods you have on hand for each environment. First look for Real Foods and whether there is a variety. Make sure there are foods you like, foods that are ready to eat, and foods you need to increase in your diet. Next, check out the Borderline and Pleasure Foods that may have crept into your life—sweet snacks, desserts, processed foods, junk foods, etc. It's important to "clean house" like this frequently. It's amazing how easy it is to slip back to eating late, and poor quality/unbalanced eating. If you check up on yourself you're bound to eat better consistently.

"Nothing can work damage to me except myself. The harm that I sustain I carry about with me and never am a real sufferer except by my own fault."

St. Bernard

Food for Thought: You'll eat what's available.

DAY FIVE
Key Theme: INSIGHT
UNDERSTANDING OBESITY

*Not* eating causes obesity—not eating well, not eating enough, and not eating on time. The cure for obesity is the reverse. Eating well (excellent food), eating enough (satisfying your hunger), and eating on time (when you first get hungry), will gradually cause weight loss and ultimately lead to natural slimness.

The concept is almost simple enough for a child to understand, but it is not an easy thing to do. It requires much more than insight. In order to make this concept work for you, you must change. Inside and out, you must change your whole approach to your diet and your eating habits. Your new understanding will provide the ongoing motivation for change. And your newfound freedom from hunger will eliminate the tendency to go back to the old ways of eating and thinking.

"Very little is needed to make a happy life. It is all within yourself, in your way of thinking."

Marcus Aurelius

Food for Thought: *Not* eating causes obesity.

DAY SIX
Key Theme: LOVE
COMPASSION FOR YOURSELF, OTHERS

Once you understand obesity, you'll begin to see how helpless people really are when they don't understand it. If you don't know what's wrong, how can you fix it? And as we all know, the traditional diet "cure" has ironically been the cause of obesity for many people besides you and me.

First, stop blaming yourself for getting fat. Next, resolve to forgive yourself for gorging, binging, starving, and gaining weight. That should be fairly easy since your efforts were made in good faith as you attempted to solve your weight problem. You didn't understand, and you weren't really in control. So forget it.

Finally, think of all the people you've secretly judged for their poor self-control. Think of them now with understanding.

"It is surely better to pardon too much than to condemn to much."
George Eliot

Food for Though: To understand is to gain compassion.

DAY SEVEN
Key Theme: DISCIPLINE
CRAVINGS AND WILLPOWER

There's a difference between normal willpower and abnormal or superhuman willpower. In order to effectively handle your sure-to-come cravings for Borderline and Pleasure Foods, you'll only need to have the normal type of willpower. Why? Because you will only let yourself get normally hungry. Remember, it's *excessive* hunger that leads to overeating.

You will avoid excess hunger like the plague it is. You will not starve yourself or go hungry very long. Consequently, you will not need to binge to catch up. You will discover, as I did, that you really do possess a fair share of self-control, and you will gladly use it to choose your diet and your eating habits wisely.

"I would have you consider your judgment and your appetite as you would two loved guests in your house. Surely you would not honor one guest above the other; for he who is more mindful of one loses the love and faith of both."

Kahlil Gibran

Food for Thought: Normal hunger, normal willpower.

DAY EIGHT
Key Theme: FREEDOM
TRYING NEW THINGS

New things, new experiences, new ideas and new approaches to old things all have something besides their newness in common. They all usually get people to react. Some people react with fear and defense, others with interest and excitement. The same newness can evoke two extreme reactions in two different people. The difference is in the people.

The novel ideas in this book and every new experience that lies before you as a result of these ideas has the potential to enrich your life. How deep and enduring the effect depends on you—how you choose to react and respond. Of course, how you respond depends on who you are. If you don't especially like yourself or your response patterns, you can change. Just decide who you want to be. Then decide how you want to react. And do it.

"The greatest discovery of my generation is that human beings can alter their lives by altering their attitudes of mind."

William James

Food for Thought: Try something new for a change in you.

DAY NINE
Key Theme: FAITH
FUEL-NEED SIGNALS

What exactly are your individual fuel needs? Only your body knows for sure. Oh, your doctor or a nutritionist might give you a general idea of the fuel on which you could get along. But even their bodies know a lot more than they do about their individual fuel needs. How can you find out more about these physiological needs and how to satisfy them? By listening carefully to your body's fuel-need signals. By trusting your body.

Listen and think. Listen when your body is just whispering the signal. Don't wait until it has to scream. By then you will be very uncomfortable. Invite your body to tell you what it needs. Treat it like a friend, and it will become one. Is there anything you can get your body just now?" Is there a quiet need you could help satisfy?

"It is the privilege of wisdom to listen."

O. W. Holmes

Food for Thought: Tune in to you body's signals—all of them.

DAY TEN
Key Theme: HOPE
PERMANENT WEIGHT LOSS

Once you have stayed off the Feast or Famine Cycle for a period of time—your body knows how much time as long as you keep eating very well and on time—you will begin a gradual, irregular descent on the scale. Some people seem to be able to lose steadily at a clip of a few pounds a month overall. Most are not so predictable, losing nothing for two months, gaining the next month then suddenly going down eight pounds the month after that. Remember that no weight loss will happen if you stay on the Cycle so be persistent in eating well and staying tune in to your hunger and fullness signals.

Some bodies are more resistant to change, and the wait to start losing is sometimes long—up to twelve months for some very famine sensitive ones. As long as they are securely off the Feast or Famine Cycle, the challenge for them is to stick to the basics and not get sloppy. If there is a long wait, you must wait. What else can you do? Want to go back to dieting?

"All human wisdom is summed up in two words—wait and hope."
Alexandre Dumas

Food for Thought: Permanent weight loss is slow, period.

DAY ELEVEN
Key Theme: SKILL
BALANCE IN EATING

Review the introduction to food categories and the Real Foods list. Jot down on paper what you ate yesterday. Don't labor over it and don't bother with amounts. You want to check balance, not calories. Now classify each food you ate into one of the four food groups in the Real Foods list. (i.e. dairy, grains, etc.). Is any group completely missing? Any group over-represented? Are fresh fruits and fresh vegetables rare or missing at times? (The foods you can eat without any concern about balance are fruits and vegetables.)

Start a shopping list to fill in the gaps. Keep balance in mind when you order a meal out. Put fresh fruits out where you can see them at home and/or at the office. In the car carry portable foods you tend to miss. Be creative. There are a thousand ways to achieve balance and some very important rewards!

"Habit is a cable; we weave a thread of it every day and at last we cannot break it."

Horace Mann

Food for Thought: Quality and variety *plus* balance.

DAY TWELVE
Key Theme: INSIGHT
NEEDING FAT

The main reason people who diet the old way go crazy, binge, and crave all the wrong foods is their need for fat. They unknowingly create this physiological (not psychological) need by going hungry or under eating much of the time. The forced calorie limitations of all diets cause biochemical changes that eventually demand extra food to promote survival fat storage. This is the mystery behind overeating (binging), cravings for fat-producing foods, preoccupation with food, depressed metabolism and fatigue—all symptoms universally experienced by dieters.

We are indeed "fearfully and wonderfully made," and we'd better seek to understand our bodies or we risk never becoming the best we can be.

"Nature imitates herself: A grain thrown into good ground brings forth fruit: a principle thrown into a good mind brings forth fruit. Everything is created and conducted by the same Master—the root, the branch, the fruits—the principles, the consequences."

Blaise Pascal

Food for Thought: Do I still *need* fat?

DAY THIRTEEN
Key Theme: LOVE
SEL-ESTEEM AND BODY IMAGE

Obesity holds people back. It can keep them half-down much of the time. It often prevents its victims from really believing in themselves. Obesity is a thief. It can rob people of their self-esteem. This is why I so desperately sought a way out for myself. I was being held back. I was half-down—I wasn't able to really believe in myself because I was fat. The fatness itself didn't really cripple me. How I felt about being fat did it.

This is true of just about every fat person everywhere. Don't be fooled. Almost no one escapes the negative self-image effects of obesity. No one is really content with his or her fatness, not even the rich and famous.

There is a way out of this burden for you. It begins with understanding but quickly leads to how you feel about yourself and your body. As you make the right choices in the kitchen, choose your attitudes towards your body wisely, too.

"If you want things to be different, perhaps the answer is to become different yourself. Become a self-believer."

Norman Vincent Peale

Food for Thought: I accept all of me.

DAY FOURTEEN
Key Theme: DISCIPLINE
PLEASURE FOOD

There is nothing wrong with Pleasure Foods. They alone don't cause obesity, and eliminating them by itself, won't cure it either. Why list them? Why even mention Pleasure Foods if there's nothing inherently wrong with them?

Pleasure Foods are just fine for fun. The trouble lies with the dieter or reckless eater who misuses them. There are two main reasons why they are misused. First, the dieter is over hungry and craves fat-producing Pleasure Foods because dieting creates the need to store extra fat. Second, all too often when hunger strikes, Pleasure Foods are available and real foods are not. That's it in a nutshell. Now go do something about it.

"A man full-fed refuses honey, but even bitter food tastes sweet to a hungry man."

Proverbs

Food for Thought: Real food for a real body.

DAY FIFTEEN
Key Theme: FREEDOM
OTHER PEOPLE PRESSURES

It takes a great deal of self-assuredness to withstand the critical eye or voice of another. There will be many difficult moments for the person who embarks on this program because of the general belief that fat people shouldn't eat very much, if at all. For some, this will be the hardest part of the program. These people have carefully avoided eating in front of anyone much of the time. They have become closet eaters. They are very sensitive to rejection and criticism and have a strong need to be accepted. Are you in this group? You will need courage.

"Whatever you do, you need courage. Whatever course you decide upon, there is always someone to tell you, you are wrong. There are always difficulties that arise which tempt you to believe that your critics are right. To map out a course of action, and follow it to an end requires some of the same courage which a soldier needs. Peace has its victories, but it takes brave men (and women) to win them."

Ralph Waldo Emerson

Food for Thought: I don't eat for other people.

DAY SIXTEEN
Key Theme: FAITH
CLOTHES: STYLE AND COMFORT

You might be thinking, *what do clothes have to do with faith?* Good question.

I used to wear tight, uncomfortable clothes, especially pants, when I was dieting. I was using the tight clothes to remind myself just how fat I was getting. This would, I imagined, curtail my eating. And I was also punishing my body for its willful appetite. Somehow, I thought, if I was in pain I would work harder to avoid eating. So much for the psychological aspects of obesity. The faith part comes in when you understand why you are still overweight and, further, what you must do to change that. You realize that discomfort will only work against you. You see that your body is not to blame and that punishing it will only backfire. So you find the most attractive and comfortable outfits you can and you wear them in good faith.

"In nature there are neither rewards nor punishments—there are consequences."

Robert G. Ingersoll

Food for Thought: I can look and feel better *now*.

DAY SEVENTEEN
Key Theme: HOPE
PLATEAUS/WAITING

One of the goals of this program is to distract the chronic dieter. A major side effect of traditional dieting is a terrible preoccupation with eating and weight, do's and don'ts. This adds to the dieter's defeat because, coupled with chronic hunger, waiting and watching for weight loss to happen creates a restlessness and impatience. "I'm suffering, I'm struggling, and I'm following all the rules. C'mon, where's my reward?" And the reward—weight loss—does come. And it goes.

The rewards of this program are immediate although the weight loss is not. For me the next best thing to getting thin was the freedom to think about other things, even while I was still overweight. I let my body decide when to eat and how much and I just stuck with keeping the food quality consistently high. This way, I was able to concentrate on my life, my work, my family and friends.

"The secret of patience is doing something else in the meanwhile."

Apples of Gold

Food for Thought: Am I distracted?

DAY EIGHTEEN
Key Theme: SKILL
HUNGER IN DISGUISE

You are learning so much about your body these first few weeks! Perhaps you've been surprised a few times—when you get hungry, what you get hungry for, how much, how little you want or need to eat. It takes a considerable amount of trust in your body to keep on satisfying its fuel-need signals when you've been taught to override them for so long. But remember, as you satisfy your body, its needs will change. Your body will need the same thing you need—to use up extra fat.

If you are uncertain about a signal your body sends, ask yourself, *does any real food sound appealing? Does food suddenly look good to me?* If you answer yes to either question, try eating some Real Food. You will soon discover whether or not you got the signal right.

"In today's thin world, our best chance is for the facts about fat to replace the myths about obesity."
From "Fat Chance in a Thin World," NOVA Program #1007

Food for Thought: When in doubt, ask yourself questions—think .

DAY NINETEEN
Key Theme: INSIGHT
FATIGUE AND OTHER BODY NEEDS

Sometimes you may feel hungry when you have another physical need. Perhaps you are overtired or nervous or dehydrated. Dehydration is a notorious mimic of hunger. Stay well hydrated to keep these two signals straight. It is not uncommon to mix up body need signals but as long as you keep your body well fed and well watered, there's no harm in mistaking its need for rest, etc. with its need for food. Sometimes we just need a break or a nap but miss these cues because we aren't thinking in those directions. Gradually, as your body becomes a bigger priority, you'll get better at knowing your body's signals and satisfying them accurately.

"How can you come to know yourself? Never by thinking, always by doing."

Johann Wolfgang von Goethe

Food for Thought: Learn to meet the right need.

DAY TWENTY
Key Theme: LOVE
TAKING CARE OF YOURSELF—AN INVENTORY

Are you a martyr? Are you a victim? Are you waiting for someone to come along and rescue you from the sweat and strain of life? Are you into silent self-pity? Are you secretly proud of your habit of self-degradation? Do you have an exaggerated need for attention? Do you play the "Ain't-It-Awful Game" to get that attention? Are you usually prepared for the worst or are you getting ready for something good to happen? Are you taking care of yourself, or are you trying to take care of everyone else in hopes that someone will notice your sacrificial spirit and take care of you? Are you as nice to yourself as you are to a good neighbor? Did you know that you are the only one who can meet your needs and change your life in any significant way? Are you ready to succeed—or are you terrified you might?

"I'm important to me! I mean much more to me than I mean to anybody I ever knew!"

The Unsinkable Molly Brown

Food for Thought: I am getting ready for success. I deserve it.

DAY TWENTY-ONE
Key Theme: DISCIPLINE
EMOTIONAL EATING AND HABIT

There is some comfort in eating, but there is no comfort in being fat. Don't forget that. There are comforts in other activities as well, and I urge you to investigate them for your personal use.

Comforting activities can be directed toward others or toward ourselves—talking with a friend, helping someone out, going for a walk, sending a card, reading a good book. Remind yourself today that so-called emotionally inspired eating is intimately related to the Feast or Famine Cycle. Getting off the Cycle should curtail the "refrigerator response" significantly, but habit may also play a role. So, if you find yourself in the kitchen asking yourself what you're hungry for and the answer is love, that what you should have. It's up to you to get or give some.

"Great battles are really won before they are actually fought. To control our passions we must govern our habits, and keep watch over ourselves in the small details of everyday life."

Sir John Lubbock

Food for Thought: The first step in breaking a habit is to think about it.

DAY TWENTY-TWO
Key Theme: FREEDOM
EATING OUT

I usually eat some real food just before going out to eat so I'll be comfortable enough to enjoy myself and alert enough to order intelligently. I used to save up my appetite for a meal away from home so I could eat, and overeat, without feeling too guilty.

That was a bad plan. In a restaurant, it always takes longer to get the food than you expect. So, if you're quite hungry when you go out, you'll likely be extremely hungry or starving by the time you're actually able eat something. Also, it is hard enough to order from a menu of very appealing food when you are only slightly hungry. It's a lot worse when you are starving. When you do get the food, it takes great restraint to savor and enjoy it. The natural thing to do is gobble it up as fast as you can. My advice is, dine early and eat before you go.

"It gives great glory to God for a person to live in this world using and appreciating the good things of life without care, without anxiety, and without inordinate passion."

Thomas Merton

Food for Thought: Be prepared to enjoy the *whole* experience.

DAY TWENTY-THREE
Key Theme: FAITH
SICKNESS/STRESS

Ralph Waldo Emerson wrote, "First, be a good animal." Now this quotation might puzzle you at first, but think about it. No one advises animals in the wild, which they should feed, a fever or a cold. So how do the animals know what to do when they are sick or under stress or danger? They know by their bodies' signals, and they instinctively follow them. Hunger sends them hunting for food. Nausea from a threat demands a fast. Thirst is an invitation to drink—to seek water. Satisfaction of these cues is the signal to stop. It's not complicated. Maybe that's why we humans have so much trouble with it.

"Studies with animals have found that obesity is not a naturally occurring phenomenon."

From "Fat Chance in a Thin World"
NOVA Program #1007

Food for Thought: Your body knows what it needs.

DAY TWENTY-FOUR
Key Theme: HOPE
GETTING SUPPORT

It can be very helpful for you to have another person to support you in this unconventional weight-loss experience. It is best if this person has read the book and shares a weight problem. You'll automatically have much in common.

Organize a group, however small, if you can. Regular, informal meetings and phone calls for sharing and reviewing the principles of understanding obesity from the perspective of adaptation will keep you going when changes are slow, especially at the beginning.

If you are alone in your recovery, don't worry. Many others have found their way to lasting weight loss without support from others—some report that they have even been successful at standing up to criticism. Use the books for support—to keep you on the path and remind you of the basics.

"Thou therefore which teachest another, teachest thou not thyself?
St. Paul

Food for Thought: I need support, one way or another.

DAY TWENTY-FIVE
Key Theme: SKILL
RECOGNIZING THE FEAST OR FAMINE CYCLE

There are five main checkpoints that indicate whether or not you are on the Feast or Famine Cycle. Any one of these factors can indicate a danger spot in your diet. Once you are completely off the Cycle, you should be consistently free of these symptoms:

Symptoms of the Feast or Famine Cycle

1.  Binging
2.  Excessive hunger
3.  Cravings for Pleasure Foods
4.  Urge to eat without hunger
5.  Emotional/stress overeating

If you still have some of these symptoms, review Chapter 2, 4, and 5. If you are completely symptom free, congratulations! You're in recovery. Remember you must stay off the Cycle to lose weight.

"The worst day of my life was the day I found myself out of control."
Shirley M., dieter

Food for Thought: Off the Cycle, in control.

DAY TWENTY-SIX
Key Theme: INSIGHT
SWEETS

Sugar-laden foods; pastries, dessert-type foods, and sugar-based drinks are very poor quality and definitely contribute to weight problems and the host of complications of obesity. The question to ask is *why* these foods are so popular in spite of their danger to people's health? It is because we are a society of dieters and reckless eaters—going hungry is common in our fast-paced lifestyle. So many of us are over hungry, and we naturally crave Pleasure Food to satisfy our biological need for sugar and fat. So, I'd have to blame the traditional quick-weight loss diets, and the very poor eating patterns of non-dieters for the preference so many have for Pleasure Foods. It's not the food that directly causes obesity. It is the powerful biology behind the need for make-up eating.

"Overweight is seldom just desserts."

Food for Thought: Real food is good for the sweet tooth.

DAY TWENTY-SEVEN
Key Theme: LOVE
BEFRIENDING YOUR BODY

It is important that you make friends with your body before you get slim.

If you dislike or even hate someone at the outset of a conversation, how much understanding are you likely to achieve? How much cooperation? How much compromise? On the other hand, if you talk with a trusted friend, someone you love and respect, there will certainly be understanding, cooperation and acceptance between you. You will even be more likely to share goals.

Accept and understand your body—its needs, its rhythms, its uniqueness. Your body needs your help to adapt healthfully to a new food environment. It absolutely depends on your choices. If you respect its needs and choose with discipline and commitment, your body will repay you with a wonderful gift.

"For without words, in friendship, all thoughts, all desires, all expectations are born and shared, with joy that is unacclaimed."

Kahlil Gibran

Food for Thought: Your body is your friend indeed.

DAY TWENTY-EIGHT
Key Theme: DISCIPLINE
EXERCISE

Exercise is said to be the component that can make or break the success of a diet program. It is true that regular exercise on the part of a dieter reflects to some extent her degree of commitment to getting in shape. But exercise, by itself, does not determine whether or not a person wins at losing. There are other very important things to consider.

Certainly, regular physical activity has many health benefits. The question for you is not whether to exercise, but how to fit the best form of exercise into your lifestyle.

You know what to do. Just do it—and often!

"I'm . . .what's known as an athletic fat person."
    Ray G. "Fat Chance in a Thin World" NOVA Program #1007

Food for Thought: I can easily fit physical activity into my life. I just have to decide to do it, and keep on deciding to do it.

DAY TWENTY-NINE
Key Theme: FREEDOM
FORGETTING THE SCALE

Some dieters don't weigh themselves. They're afraid to because they feel—and are—so out of control at times. They figure the numbers probably are too. The negative experiences they have had all their dieting lives have conditioned them to avoid standing on the scale. For some, it is almost a phobia.

Most dieters are just the opposite. They weigh themselves compulsively, even many times a day. They want to know, to be reassured, to feel more in control of their weight. This extreme is also fear-motivated.

Once you turn your diet controls over to your body, with the exception of food quality, you will need neither escape nor reassurance from the scale. You will know, as you provide of great food on demand for your body each day, that in time, you will be the perfect weight for you.

"I'm not overweight, I'm under tall."

Garfield

Food for Thought: Getting thin isn't a numbers game.

DAY THIRTY
Key Theme: FAITH
LETTING GO

I hope by now you're getting on nicely with the rest of your life. Stay busy! Do new things! There is so much more to your life than your physical shape. And as you grow slowly thinner naturally, you will discover that more of your real self will be free to emerge. You may even be surprised at the new you! Frankly, I am a better person since I stopped dieting and learned to eat like a normal person. I suspect that you will be, too.

"Therefore I bid you put away anxious thought about food and drink to keep you alive, and clothes to cover your body. Surely life is more than food, the body more than clothes."

Jesus

Food for thought: I'm getting better—all of me.

DAY THIRTY-ONE
Key Theme: HOPE
IMAGING SUCCESS

There is a term used in psychology that I love. It is Creative Anticipation, and it refers to the fact that what we deeply expect to happen usually does. Whether or not you believe this does not alter its profound reality. The power in this truth lies in the fact that our beliefs affect our behaviors. And behaviors—including our choices—certainly influence what happens to us, what course our life takes.

So fill your thoughts with images of what you want to be and what you hope to accomplish. Reject doubt and fear. Hang on to your vision for yourself. Hold the image of your ideal life firmly in your mind and don't let go.

"Because a thing seems difficult for you, do not think it is impossible for anyone to accomplish. But whatever is possible for another, believe that you, too, are capable of it."

Marcus Aurelius

Food for thought: I will succeed and accomplish my dreams.

BEYOND THIRTY-ONE DAYS: OWNING YOUR RECOVERY

This is a challenging program—not for easily discouraged or self-pitying types. It takes perseverance and determination—faith and patience.

# READER'S GUIDE

Chapter 1

1. How have various diets hooked you into thinking they were "different?"
2. What was your reaction to the idea that excess body fat is a "positive" adaptation?
3. When you are not dieting, do you try to control your eating anyway?
4. What was your very first diet? How overweight were you?
5. Do you habitually "eat late?"
6. When you get in touch with your hunger, are you often famished or starving?

Chapter 2

1. Can you describe the war you have been in with your body as a dieter?
2. What part of the feast or famine cycle do you relate to the most?
3. Can you see the role that Denial has played in your feast or famine diet cycle?
4. Do you accept the 95% long-term failure rate for traditional quick weight loss diets?

5. Is the idea of losing weight quickly and keeping it off something you still hope to accomplish?

## Chapter 3

1. What is your Famine Sensitivity? How can knowing about this help you change?
2. Do you believe you're addicted to food? Has this diagnosis helped you understand your eating behavior in the past?
3. Have you ever experienced an "emotionally triggered" binge? After reading about emotional eating, what do you think might have really happened?
4. When you are dieting, what types of foods do you crave? Have you blamed food addiction, carbohydrate addiction, or sugar addiction in the past?

## Chapter 4

1. When did you first get out of touch with your hunger?
2. Does the idea of eating whenever you get hungry scare you?
3. Have you ever used any appetite suppressants? What was their overall effect?
4. Do you consider yourself to be always hungry or never hungry?
5. Do you believe that your hunger and fullness signals can actually become normal?

## Chapter 5

1. What do you think about when someone says "diet?"
2. Have you ever thought of calories as good for you?
3. What was the first thing you thought when you read the Real Food List?
4. Does the engine fuel analogy help you prioritize different foods?

5. How is your food availability coming along?

## Chapter 6

1. Are you still confidant that you are an emotional overeater—and that you eat for comfort?
2. Do you see similarities between your diet cycles and the bears' hibernation cycles?
3. Have you ever tried behavior modification techniques in your weight loss efforts?
4. Did the TV programs about enormous, rapid weight loss ever appeal to your hopes?
5. What do you think about fast weight loss schools for kids?

## Chapter 7

1. How long have you been at war with your body? Are you ready to make peace?
2. Do you think it's possible for you to stop eating and overeating at night?
3. How much cooperation are you likely to get at home? Will sabotage be a problem?
4. What do you think is a realistic goal weight for you? How did you arrive at that number?

## Chapter 8

1. Are you feeling overwhelmed by this program's emphasis on personal responsibility?
2. Were you surprised by the idea that exercise isn't necessarily a great tool for weight loss?
3. Name three habits you have developed. How did they become your habits?

4. Where can you expand your every day lifestyle to include spurts of activity?
5. Would it be possible for you to learn to cook very simple meals, and order simple items at a restaurant?

## Chapter 9

1. Does the lack of structure of this approach appeal to you or worry you?
2. Is the idea of "speeding it up" remind you of dieting to lose weight faster?
3. How does five years to lose weight sound compared to six months?
4. What do you think will be your biggest challenges on this program? Do you believe you can you overcome these obstacles?
5. Do these principles give you hope of learning to eat and live like a normal person?

# INDEX

## D

## E

# F

Famine  6, 7, 8, 15, 18, 19, 20, 21,
22, 25, 27, 28, 29, 31, 32, 35,
36, 37, 38, 39, 40, 41, 42, 43,
48, 49, 55, 56, 58, 59, 60, 61,
62, 64, 65, 74, 77, 78, 79, 81,
84, 85, 88, 89, 90, 94, 97,
100, 101, 102, 103, 104, 107,
108, 115, 120, 121, 122, 126,
127, 128, 129, 131, 132, 133,
134, 135, 136, 137, 138, 141,
142, 143, 145, 146, 147, 148,
149, 150, 152, 153, 154, 160,
165, 166, 168, 169, 170, 172,
173, 179, 180, 181, 184, 186,
189, 193, 198, 200, 209, 210
Famine sensitivity  32, 35, 39, 40,
41, 42, 43, 94, 107, 108, 115,
121, 122, 133, 169, 210
Fat  1, 2, 4, 5, 6, 7, 8, 9, 10, 11, 13,
14, 15, 17, 18, 19, 23, 25, 26,
27, 28, 29, 32, 33, 34, 35, 36,
38, 40, 41, 42, 43, 46, 49,
54, 55, 56, 58, 59, 63, 64, 67,
69, 70, 71, 73, 74, 76, 78, 81,
82, 83, 89, 94, 96, 97, 102,
103, 104, 105, 106, 112, 113,
120, 121, 124, 129, 131, 134,
136, 138, 142, 143, 144, 146,
148, 153, 154, 155, 160, 161,
164, 167, 168, 169, 171, 172,
174, 175, 177, 180, 209
Fat storage  6, 25, 102, 103, 121,
134, 168, 169

Fear of famines  134
Feast or famine cycle  31, 35, 37,
39, 56, 58, 59, 60, 61, 62, 65,
74, 77, 78, 79, 81, 84, 85, 88,
89, 97, 102, 103, 107, 108,
120, 122, 126, 127, 128, 129,
131, 132, 134, 135, 136, 137,
138, 141, 142, 143, 145, 146,
147, 149, 150, 152, 153, 154,
160, 165, 166, 168, 170, 172,
173, 179, 180, 181, 186, 193,
200, 209
Food  iii, v, xi, xv, 3, 5, 6, 7, 8, 9,
10, 11, 12, 13, 14, 15, 16, 17,
18, 21, 22, 24, 25, 26, 27, 28,
29, 31, 32, 33, 34, 35, 38, 40,
41, 42, 43, 44, 45, 46, 47, 49,
50, 54, 55, 56, 57, 58, 59, 60,
61, 62, 63, 64, 65, 66, 67, 68,
69, 70, 71, 72, 73, 74, 75, 76,
77, 78, 79, 80, 81, 82, 83, 84,
85, 86, 87, 88, 89, 90, 91,
94, 95, 96, 97, 98, 99, 100,
101, 102, 103, 104, 105, 107,
108, 109, 110, 111, 112, 113,
119, 121, 122, 123, 124, 125,
126, 127, 129, 130, 131, 132,
134, 136, 137, 138, 139, 140,
141, 142, 143, 144, 145, 146,
147, 148, 149, 150, 151, 152,
153, 154, 155, 159, 160, 161,
162, 163, 164, 165, 166, 167,
168, 169, 170, 171, 172, 173,
174, 176, 177, 179, 180, 181,
182, 183, 184, 185, 187, 189,

# About the Author

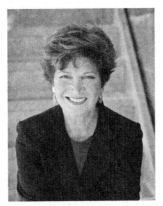

*Lisa Buth Photography*

Obesity and eating disorders specialist Jean Antonello was trapped in the yo-yo diet cycle for seventeen years before she discovered a startling fact: She was fighting a war against her body she could not win. Desperate to find lasting weight loss, she turned to her nursing education for a solution. The fundamentals she learned there helped her see dieting from a new perspective—as threat to her survival. Armed with these new insights, Jean began to cooperate with her body instead of battling it, and finally lost weight for good. Knowing countless others had tried and failed as she had, Jean embarked on a mission to share her discoveries with frustrated dieters everywhere. She has been coaching and writing about her Naturally Thin® principles since 1990, with three books on the subject: *How to Become Naturally Thin by Eating More, Breaking Out of Food Jail* and *Naturally Thin Kids. NATURALLY THIN* is a compilation of her groundbreaking work, written to reach even more people with this liberating information.

www.naturally-thin.com

CPSIA information can be obtained
at www.ICGtesting.com
Printed in the USA
LVOW13s1030141117

556239LV00014B/251/P